Sex Endocrinology

FIRST EDITION

A HANDBOOK
FOR THE MEDICAL
AND ALLIED
PROFESSIONS

Schering Corporation

MEDICAL RESEARCH DIVISION

BLOOMFIELD, N. J.

1945

ISSUED BY THE SCHERING CORPORATION · MEDICAL RESEARCH DIVISION · COPR. 1944

$Foreword$: Twenty years ago, the science of endocrinology was in its infancy, and endocrine diagnosis relied completely upon the simple recounting of symptoms and a physical examination. Hormone therapy was crude and highly inefficient; and such prognoses as were occasionally hazarded varied with the individual clinician's enthusiasms. In the short space of a decade, however, endocrinology — and more specifically its most elusive subdivision, sex endocrinology — has made enormous strides. Today, the clinician has at his command diagnostic criteria and objective tests permitting relatively accurate diagnosis and effective therapy in most cases.

In the growth of the new science, chemistry has played a most important part, and to it must be credited the availability of the pure crystalline hormones which make possible the dramatic rehabilitation of sex hormone deficient subjects. And because the pure hormones are available today in exactly the same form as elaborated in the body, a better understanding of their true role is possible. Thus, it is, that the ovarian and testicular hormones have been found to be more than "sex hormones". Their effects on the human organism are many, and encompass, in addition to their obvious uses, such diverse actions as regulation of personality, and metabolism.

The story of the sex hormones, their effects on the generative tract, as well as other body functions, and their relation to good health is an absorbing one. This story is told in the following pages with the hope that it may contribute to a better understanding of the function of the sex hormones as applied in modern therapeutics.

CONTENTS

CHAPTER ONE

INTRODUCTION TO ENDOCRINOLOGY

Man has been fascinated by sex from the earliest times. The primitive cave drawings of sexual organs, the phallic statues of African gods, the ornamental drawings of the sex act found on the walls of buried Pompeii, and, in more recent times, the surprisingly accurate anatomic sketches of Leonardo da Vinci—all testify to the appreciation of the role of sex in the daily life of man.

The external differences between man and woman were apparent to even the earliest human inhabitants of this globe. The reasons for these differences must certainly have been less evident, for centuries elapsed before primitive people realized the relationship between sexual intercourse and birth.

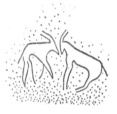

The perpetuation of the species is the ultimate aim of the differentiation into male and female, and of the endowment of men and women with special characteristics and organs. In the course of development, man came to know more and more about himself and his bodily functions, and the mystery of sex began slowly to unfold. But it was not until recently, with the discovery of the sex hormones, that scientists began to understand better the essential physiological differences between man and woman.

The story of the sex hormones is an absorbing chapter in the history of science. But, first, a few words about hormones in general.

HORMONES AND ENDOCRINE GLANDS

Hormones (G., *hormao*, arouse) are chemical substances which are prepared by groups of specialized body cells, known as endocrine (G., *endon*, within + *krino*, separate) glands. These endocrine glands, really small chemical laboratories, extract materials from the blood stream and convert them into hormones, which are then secreted directly into the blood stream and carried to every living body cell. Since the hormones are poured into the blood without passing through an excretory canal or duct, these glands are also called glands of internal secretion or ductless glands. Endocrinology is the study of the endocrine glands and the hormones that they produce.

> Another group of glands is known as the glands of external secretion or exocrine (G., *exo*, out of + *krino*, separate) glands, because their secretions are eliminated through ducts, and are usually utilized for specialized functions in a particular region rather than throughout the entire body. Examples of external secretions are perspiration, saliva, gastric juice, etc.

Location

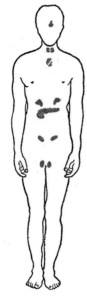

LOCATION OF ENDOCRINE GLANDS

The different endocrine glands are situated in various parts of the body. The pituitary gland, for instance, is within the skull; the thyroid and parathyroid glands, in the neck; the pancreas,* the adrenals and the ovaries, in the abdomen; and the testicles, in the scrotum. The hormones secreted by these glands have specific functions, which may be exerted far from their place of origin. For this reason, they have been called "chemical messengers".

---

*The pancreas is a mixed gland because it contains both endocrine and exocrine portions: the endocrine secretion, insulin, passes directly into the blood; the exocrine secretion, the pancreatic juice (containing digestive enzymes), is excreted through the pancreatic duct into the small intestine.

Importance

Certain hormones, such as those secreted by the adrenal cortex, are absolutely essential to life. The deficiency of other hormones, such as thyroxin, secreted by the thyroid, while not absolutely necessary for the maintenance of life, results in diminished physical and mental activity, incompatible with *normal* existence. Still others, such as the sex hormones, secreted by the gonads* (G., *gonē*, seed), are essential both for full health and the production of new life.

Interrelationship

The pituitary gland, about the size of an acorn, is situated at the base of the brain. It contains three lobes: anterior, intermediary and posterior.

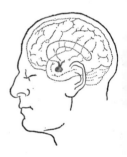

LOCATION OF PITUITARY

The anterior pituitary controls the activities of all the endocrine glands—it is truly the "master gland", the conductor of the hormonal symphony. In the normal body, there is a harmonious interrelationship between the endocrine glands. In the same way as an orchestral instrument "off beat" may disturb the performance of another instrumentalist, abnormal function of a particular endocrine gland may cause disturbed function of another gland. The various glands of internal secretion respond to the stimulus of the anterior pituitary and are influenced by other endocrine glands. These, in turn, influence the anterior pituitary.

EARLY ENDOCRINOLOGY

Primitive man attributed great virtues to the internal organs obtained from slain enemies or animals. The warrior

---

*Gonad is a general term for sex gland—the female gonad is the ovary and the male gonad is the testicle. The ovary produces ova (plural of L., *ovum*, egg) and the two female hormones. The testicle produces spermatozoa (plural of spermatozoon, from G., *sperma*, seed + *zoon*, animal) and the male hormone.

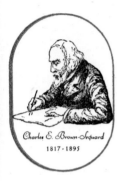

Charles E. Brown-Sequard
1817-1895

sought to increase his courage by eating the heart of his adversary and to heighten his sexual powers by partaking of his enemy's testicles.

It is indeed a far cry from such mystical and magical beliefs to the modern science of endocrinology. And yet, as late as 1889, Brown-Sequard, a famous French physiologist, at the age of 72, treated himself for waning vigor with injections of aqueous extracts of testicles of dogs and guineapigs. It is highly improbable, for reasons that will presently appear, that the spectacular rejuvenation that he reported was due to anything more than autosuggestion.

Brown-Sequard, and others before him, were right in assuming that the male sex principle is produced in the testicle. However, though the male hormone occurs in the testes, and, similarly, the female hormone in the ovaries, they are present in exceedingly minute quantities at any one moment, because they are not stored there but are secreted into the blood stream almost as soon as they are produced. In fact, it has been calculated that it would require about a quarter of a ton of bull testicles by injection to furnish an average dose of male sex hormone, and over 300 pounds of sow ovaries by injection to furnish an adequate dose of the female sex hormone.

Realizing the inertness of almost all glandular material taken by mouth, investigators prepared aqueous extracts of the testes and ovaries. These extracts, similar to those employed by Brown-Sequard, were administered by injection but proved inert since the sex hormones are insoluble in water and are best administered in oil solvents. The solubility of the sex hormones and other physical and chemical properties can best be understood by a consideration of their chemical structure.

CHAPTER TWO

CHEMISTRY OF THE SEX HORMONES

On the basis of chemical and physiological differences, the sex hormones are classified in three groups:

1. The estrogenic hormone group (female hormone).
2. The corpus luteum hormone group (female hormone).
3. The androgenic hormone group (male hormone).

STEROIDS

Although the actions of these hormones differ widely, their basic chemical structure is quite similar in the possession of a common nucleus known as the steroid (G., *stereos*, solid + *eidos*, similar) nucleus. Minor differences in their molecular structure, such as the number of double-bonds and the presence of side-chains, account for the striking differences in biological activity of the sex hormones or sex steroids, as they are also called. In addition to the sex hormones, the steroid nucleus occurs widely in other physiological substances, such as the bile acids, the active principles of the digitalis glucosides, and the hormones of the adrenal cortex.

The steroids include another group of natural substances, the sterols (G., *stereos*, solid + Chem., *ol*, alcohol), which occur in animal and plant fats, and oils. Cholesterol is the characteristic sterol of the higher animal organism. Another important sterol is vitamin D.

It is thus apparent that the sex hormones are natural sub-stances, related to the wide-spread sterols, and are among the basic constituents of living cells.

THE STEROID NUCLEUS

The structure of complex organic compounds, such as the sex hormones, can be understood by means of successive simple steps.

Starting with benzene, condensation with another benzene ring results in naphthalene.

If still another benzene ring is added, the result is phenan-threne. The hydrogenation of phenanthrene results in per-hydrophenanthrene.

If finally, a 5-carbon ring is added, perhydro-cyclopenteno-phenanthrene is obtained. This is the steroid nucleus, which is customarily written in abbreviated form, as:

This nucleus recurs with minor changes in the various sex hormones and also in the excretion forms of the hormones.

After the sex hormones have been utilized by the body, they are broken down and eliminated, usually in the urine. Although some of these excretion products differ from the original hormones only slightly in chemical structure, they are all markedly less active and most of them are physiologically inert.

THE ESTROGENIC HORMONE GROUP

Estrogen (G., *oistros*, mad desire + *gennao*, produce) or estrogenic hormones are responsible for the changes occurring in the reproductive organs of female animals during the mating season (heat, rut or estrus).

The principal estrogen is alpha-estradiol (Fig. I). It is also known as the follicular hormone because it is obtained from the follicles of the ovary. After performing its function in the body, alpha-estradiol is eliminated in the urine as estrone (Fig. II) and estriol (Fig. III).

In keeping with the general rule that the primary hormone is always more active than its excretion forms, it has been found that alpha-estradiol is approximately 12 times more potent than estrone and at least 80 times more potent than estriol. As will be seen in the formulae, these wide differences in biological activity depend upon comparatively slight variations in chemical structure.

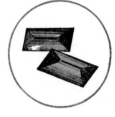

ALPHA-ESTRADIOL
CRYSTALS

Fig. I   Fig. II   Fig. III

Since alpha-estradiol (PROGYNON-DH)* is rapidly absorbed and immediately effective when injected, attempts were made to prolong its therapeutic effect in order to imitate the steady, continuous action of a functioning gland. It was found that various esters of alpha-estradiol produced prolonged action because they were hydrolyzed slowly in the tissues. The most active of these is the benzoate, providing an intensity and duration of action well suited to intramuscular injection. The dipropionate, though less potent, is employed to obtain a somewhat more prolonged effect.

THE CORPUS LUTEUM HORMONE GROUP

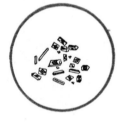

PROGESTERONE CRYSTALS

The corpus luteum hormone and its derivatives are called progestins (L., *pro*, in favor of + *gestatio*, from gestare, to bear) because they are directly concerned with pregnancy and its successful completion. The pure, crystalline hormone (PROLUTON) is known chemically as progesterone, or pregnenedione (Fig. IV), and is employed medically by injection. It is not excreted in the urine as such but as a biologically inactive derivative, pregnandiol.

The orally effective progestin (PRANONE) is pregneninolon or anhydrohydroxy-progesterone (Fig. V).

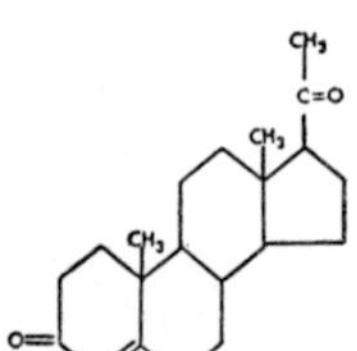

Fig. IV

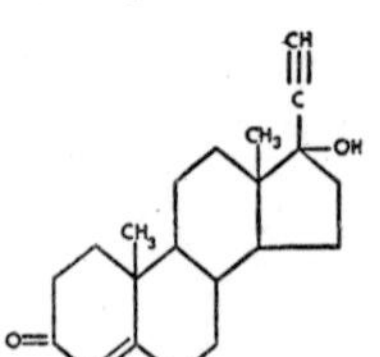

Fig. V

*Alpha-estradiol (PROGYNON-DH) is employed orally and also in ointment form locally whenever a direct, local effect is desired. Alpha-estradiol benzoate (PROGYNON-B) and the alpha-estradiol dipropionate (PROGYNON-DP) are employed only by injection.

As its name indicates, it may be considered as progesterone which has been modified by the addition of a hydroxyl radical and the elimination of a molecule of water.

When given by mouth in approximately five times the dosage of progesterone intramuscularly, it causes corpus luteum hormone effects and may be used when injections are inconvenient or impossible.

THE ANDROGENIC HORMONE GROUP

Members of this group are known as androgens (G., *andr-*, man + *gennao*, produce) because of their masculinizing properties. The principal androgen is the male sex hormone itself, testosterone or androstenolone (Fig. VI).

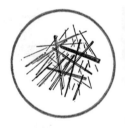

TESTOSTERONE CRYSTALS

Fig. VI   Fig. VII   Fig. VIII

Testosterone is the primary male sex hormone actually obtained from the testis and is the most potent androgen known. Clinically, it is administered as solid ORETON-F Pellets implanted subcutaneously. When testosterone is injected in solution hypodermically, its effects are rapid, but of short duration. To prolong its action in the body it is administered in an esterified form, as testosterone propionate.

Testosterone propionate (Fig. VII) is known as ORETON. It is metabolized in the body and then excreted in the urine as the less active derivatives, androsterone and dehydro*iso*-androsterone.

The orally effective androgen is methyl testosterone (Fig. VIII), ORETON-M. When given by mouth in the ratio of approximately five times the intramuscular dosage, it duplicates the clinical effects of the male sex hormone. It may also be applied in the form of an ointment, acting promptly by absorption through the skin.

SEX HORMONES AND THEIR EXCRETION PRODUCTS

FEMALE

*Estrogens**	*Progestins*
1. Alpha-estradiol or follicular hormone (PROGYNON).	1. Progesterone or corpus luteum hormone (PROLUTON).
2. Estrone ⎱ Less active urinary excretion products. 3. Estriol ⎰	2. Anhydrohydroxy-progesterone or pregneninolon (PRANONE).
	3. Pregnandiol-urinary excretion product having no biological activity.

MALE

Androgens

1. Testosterone—Testicular Hormone (ORETON)
2. Androsterone ⎱ Slightly active urinary
3. Dehydro*iso*androsterone ⎰ excretion products.

---

*The term *female* sex hormone is frequently used synonymously with estrogen, but exception may be taken to this name (as to "ovarian hormone") since a progestin or corpus luteum hormone is also an ovarian or female sex hormone.

CHAPTER THREE

HISTORY OF SEX ENDOCRINOLOGY

THE ESTROGENIC HORMONE

The analogy between the ovary and testis was stressed by early anatomists who, as late as 1555, still referred to the ovary as the "female testis". The term ovary did not come into use until a century later.

The changes following removal of the ovaries were discovered far later than those following removal of the testes. The ovaries are hidden within the abdominal cavity, and relatively safe from inquisitive marauders; while the testes, in their exposed position, could readily be removed by a comparatively simple procedure. And so it was that the effects of castration in women were not recognized until 1750. However, it took another hundred years to discover the direct relationship between the ovaries and the female sexual organs and secondary sex characteristics. Toward the end of the 19th century, ovaries were transplanted into castrated women and animals, reversing, even if only temporarily, the changes resulting from castration. Following the grafting operation, castrated women menstruated again, and castrated animals entered into heat and received the male.

Since few grafts "took", and then only temporarily, it was thought that feeding dried ovaries by mouth would effectively replace the missing ovarian tissue. During this time, "desiccated ovarian substance" and similar preparations enjoyed a considerable vogue. Their actual effects, however, were nil. Recourse was then had to injections of aqueous extracts of ovaries, but results were as dubious as those obtained by Brown-Sequard with his testicular extracts.

Matters were thus at a standstill until 1923, when Allen and Doisy succeeded in demonstrating that the follicular fluid obtained from animals' ovaries contained some èstrogenic substance, which they could not, however, identify at the time. Six years later, Doisy, Veler and Thayer, and Butenandt, obtained a crystalline estrogen from human pregnancy urine. This was named theelin (G., *thëlys*, female); and because it was an estrogenic hormone with a ketone group, it was also called estrone. A year or so later, another estrogen was obtained from urine. It was named theelol or estriol because of the presence of three hydroxyl groups.

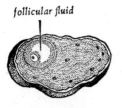

follicular fluid

MATURE OVARIAN
FOLLICLE

In 1932, Schwenk of the Schering Corporation, together with Hildebrandt, prepared a new, very potent estrogen, now known to be the primary hormone of the ovarian follicle. It was called dihydrotheelin, or alpha-estradiol, because of the presence of two hydroxyl groups ("alpha" refers to the active isomer). Three years later, MacCorquodale, Thayer and Doisy at St. Louis University, completed a 13 year investigation, during which time they painstakingly extracted the follicular fluid from four tons of sow ovaries. They succeeded in obtaining about 10 milligrams of a highly active estrogen which, by chemical and biological tests, was reported to be identical with the alpha-estradiol previously prepared by Schwenk.

It was thus shown that alpha-estradiol is the true primary follicular hormone as extracted from the follicles of the ovary, and that estrone and estriol are its excretion products.

THE CORPUS LUTEUM HORMONE

Although the presence of the corpus luteum or "yellow body" in mammalian ovaries was observed as early as 1573, its true function as an endocrine gland concerned with maintaining pregnancy was not suspected until more than three centuries later. In 1903, Fraenkel found that the removal of the corpora lutea from rabbits during early pregnancy resulted in abortion; and in 1907, Loeb demonstrated that the corpus luteum specifically prepared the uterus to receive a fertilized ovum.

And so, patients with corpus luteum deficiency were fed "desiccated corpus luteum" by mouth in the vain hope of thus replenishing the deficiency. However, only infinitesimal quantities of corpus luteum hormone are present in these inert preparations, which are ineffective even in large amounts.

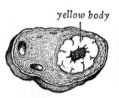

yellow body

CORPUS LUTEUM

The actual existence of a corpus luteum hormone was demonstrated in 1928 by Weichert, who produced definite progestational changes in the animal uterus with extracts from corpora lutea. The hormone was isolated in pure form in 1932 by Wintersteiner and Allen and by other investigators. In 1934, several investigators simultaneously succeeded in synthesizing it from stigmasterol (a plant sterol found in the soya bean) and from pregnandiol. It was called progesterone because of its progestational effect on the uterus, and received the -one ending because of the presence of the ketone group in its formula.

Although highly effective by injection, progesterone was found to have no action when taken by mouth. In 1938, an orally effective progestin, anhydrohydroxy-progesterone (PRANONE), was synthesized. Experimental and clinical investigation showed that it was a true progestin and, when given by mouth, duplicated the biologic effects of progesterone (PROLUTON) administered by injection.

THE MALE SEX HORMONE

It was known from most ancient times that the loss of the testicles caused marked changes in the development of the penis and other sexual organs, as well as the general appearance and behavior of the male of any species. Castration was practised on common farm animals usually for gastronomic reasons, and on human beings for religious reasons and also to produce a highly specialized type of watchman —the harem eunuch. As late as the beginning of the 20th century, castration was a religious rite among various sects, for example, the Skoptsy of Russia.

John Hunter (1792) had a clear understanding that the male sexual organs were associated with testicular activity, but he did not know that control rested upon internal secretions. The first important physiologic experiment to show how the testes influence the body was that of Berthold, who, in 1849, castrated a rooster and re-implanted the testes in other body sites. The re-implanted testicles maintained the normal sexual status of the rooster, thereby demonstrating the fact of an internal secretion for the first time. Following this classic demonstration, attempts were made to treat male deficiencies by feeding dried, powdered testes by mouth (under the resounding title of "desiccated orchic substance") or by injecting aqueous testicular extracts.

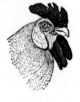

CASTRATED ROOSTER SHOWING SHRUNKEN COMB AND WATTLES

When it became apparent that these substances were completely inert, various rejuvenation procedures were attempted, such as ligation of the vas deferens (Steinach operation) and grafting of animal testicles (Voronoff operation). It was found, however, that testicular transplants from goats, dogs and monkeys did not "take"; and that ape testicles, which did "take", had temporary effects only, since they were absorbed by the body after a time. Realizing that the active male principle is definitely elaborated in the testes, investigators attempted to improve the methods of extraction. Finally, in 1927, McGee, using lipoid solvents (in which steroid hormones are soluble), succeeded in obtaining active extracts of bull testes.

Following the pioneer studies on the excretion of hormones by Aschheim and Zondek, hormones of every sort were looked for in the urine, and, to be sure, androgenic substances were found in the urine of men. These proved to be androsterone and dehydro*iso*androsterone, which were shown later to be eliminated end-products of the male sex hormone, just as estrone and estriol are elimination products of the female sex hormone.* In 1929, Koch and Gallagher obtained concentrates from bull testes which were five to ten times as potent as androsterone.

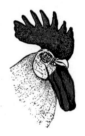

EFFECT FOLLOWING
TESTICLE IMPLANT
IN CASTRATED
ROOSTER

The male hormone itself was isolated by Laqueur in 1935, and shortly afterward, it was synthesized by Ruzicka and by Butenandt, using cholesterol as the starting material. It was called testosterone because it is the only androgen found in the testis, and received the -*one* ending because of the presence of a ketone group in its structure.

Like progesterone, testosterone was found to be effective by injection, but inactive by mouth. In 1940, an orally effective methyl derivative (ORETON-M) was made available, and for the first time, successful therapy with male sex hormone by mouth was possible.

---

*Because of their low androgenic activity, the elimination products of testosterone are no longer used in medicine.

PRESENT STATUS

Thus, it is evident that the availability of the sex hormones for clinical use is the result of a vast amount of research work. Their preparation on a large scale depends on suitable methods of synthesis which have been elaborated, in the main, within the last decade. The actual synthesis of true physiological hormones as found in the body represents the culmination of a number of previous steps in the history of endocrinology: detection, extraction, isolation, identification. The present state of knowledge, however, is still far from complete, and it is certain that the young science of sex endocrinology will continue to unlock further the mysteries of sex and also many of the problems of constitution such as general body growth, fatigue, resistance to infection, bone healing, psychic disturbances, etc.

Recently, certain unsaturated synthetic chemical compounds, such as stilbestrol and hexestrol, entirely unrelated to the natural steroid structure, have been found to have estrogenic action. These substances, however, are foreign to the body and are *not* hormones. Their clinical application is limited by certain toxic reactions, whose incidence increases with the size of the dose.

CHAPTER FOUR

SEX FUNCTION AND SEX ANATOMY

The ages of man — childhood, maturity and old age — reflect, among other things, the state of his endocrine glands and, particularly, of his sex glands.

During childhood, the sex glands are practically inactive, and the sex organs develop at a comparatively slow rate. Yet, even the small amounts of sex hormones present in children seem sufficient to insure definite differences in temperament and structure between boys and girls.

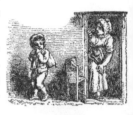

At puberty, dramatic changes take place and the whole sexual apparatus becomes active. In the boy, the voice deepens, hair begins to appear in the pubic region, on the body and on the face; the body contour becomes more angular; and masculine mental traits appear, including a deep and lively interest in the female sex. The penis develops and the adolescent boy begins to experience erections and may have ejaculations. From the point of view of the perpetuation of the species, he has attained maturity.

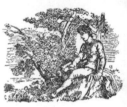

The onset of puberty in girls is even more remarkable. In addition to the feminine hair distribution and the rounded body contours, the breasts develop and menstruation begins, the latter recurring as a periodic monthly phenomenon during her entire reproductive life (except, of course, during pregnancy). The psyche of the adolescent girl becomes typically feminine, and the "wiles of Eve come unbidden to her aid". She has taken her place in Nature's great drama.

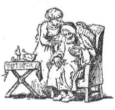

AFTER ENGRAVINGS
BY STODDARD

The transformation of the child at puberty, and his (or her) continued development during adulthood, are directly under the control of the sex hormones. Adult sexual maturity, which lasts for a fairly definite period, is followed by a period of sexual aging, during which the sex hormones diminish, the sex organs gradually atrophy and sex function declines. The tide of the hormones is on the wane, as is life itself, and the vigorous epoch of propagation has passed.

REPRODUCTION

Reproduction is a sowing and reaping — and for its successful accomplishment are needed fertile seed, sturdy implements and a receptive soil.

1. *The seed.* The spermatozoa and the ova are the germ cells whose union is necessary for the creation of new life. They are produced in the sex glands (primary sex organs or gonads) which also secrete the sex hormones. (Plate VI)

2. *The implements.* These are the accessory sex organs, which consist mainly of an elaborate system of canals and tubes for the safe transport of the germ cells from their respective places of manufacture to their rendezvous within the female. In the male, they are the epididymis, vas deferens, seminal vesicles, prostate and penis. In the female, they are the fallopian tubes, uterus, vagina, clitoris and vulva. The development of the accessory sex organs in each sex is under the direct control of their respective sex hormones.

3. *The soil.* The uterus is an accessory sex organ especially adapted to the nutrition and growth of the embryo. It undergoes periodic monthly changes which renew its lining and prepare it to receive a fertilized ovum. (Plate II)

Testes and penis in the male, and ovaries, tubes, uterus and vagina in the female are, of course, the necessary reproductive attributes of sex. There are also other factors which play a role in the reproductive drama. These are the secondary sex characteristics—bodily contour, hair distribution, voice changes, breast development, psychic traits—which appear at puberty and are responsible for the maleness of the man and the womanliness of woman, and help assure a fruitful meeting of the sexes.

The secondary sex characteristics, like the sexual organs themselves, are directly under the control of the sex hormones, and their development depends on an adequate amount of the hormones circulating in the blood. When the hormonal supply is inadequate, the individual presents varying degrees of sexual underdevelopment or hypogonadism (G., *hypo*, under + *gonē*, seed). The hypogonad male may have rounded feminine contours, high-pitched voice, feminine hair distribution, small penis, etc., and may not experience the usual pleasant sensations when contemplating the fair sex. Sexual underdevelopment in the female is usually less obvious. However, the breasts may be small, the uterus underdeveloped, and menstruation may be absent. These states are susceptible to treatment with the sex hormones. One of the proudest achievements of sex endocrinology is the ability to replace the sex hormones lacking in the body with identical ones produced in the laboratory, and thus physiologically advancing the individual to a normal sexual status. (Plates IV and VIII)

*Female Reproductive System**

OVARIES

The ovaries, two small plum-sized organs lying low in either side of the pelvis, contain thousands of minute collec-

*See Plates I and II.

tions of cells. These cell groups are called primary ovarian follicles, a number of which develop into mature (graafian) follicles. These follicles have two functions: the production of ova and the female hormones. Approximately once a month during the reproductive life of a woman, an ovum is expelled from one of the ovaries and, if fertilized, will develop into an embryo. The internal secretions of the ovary periodically prepare the uterus for pregnancy. If pregnancy does not take place, menstruation occurs. The menses have been termed the "tears of the uterus" because of the failure to conceive.

corpus luteum

graafian follicle

CROSS-SECTION OF OVARY

FALLOPIAN TUBES

The liberated ovum passes into one of the fallopian tubes, which are connecting tubes extending from the ovary to the uterus. The meeting of the ovum with a spermatozoon normally takes place in this (fallopian) tube. The ovum, fertilized or unfertilized, then goes down the tube and ultimately reaches the uterus.

UTERUS

The uterus is a hollow, muscular organ which opens below into the vagina through the cervix or neck of the uterus. It is composed of three layers that are intimately connected with each other:

1. The endometrium (G., *endon*, within + *metra*, uterus), the inner lining of the uterus, is covered by a single layer of cells and microscopic uterine glands. It undergoes changes necessary for the nesting, anchoring or nidation of the fertilized ovum, and later is devoted to the nutrition of the developing embryo.

2. The myometrium (G., *myo*, muscle + *metra*, uterus), the thick middle layer composed mainly of smooth muscle,

develops greatly during pregnancy and helps protect the embryo against injury. During labor, the delivery of the baby is carried out by its muscular contractions.

3. The serosa, the thin, outer covering of the uterus.

VAGINA

The vagina is a muscular tube especially adapted to receive the penis during intercourse and the spermatozoa following ejaculation, and is capable of great dilatation to permit the passage of the baby during delivery. It extends from the lower end of the uterus to the external genitalia (which comprise the labia majora, labia minora, clitoris, etc.). The vagina is lined by mucous membrane composed of several layers of cells, resembling the mucous membrane of the mouth or the tongue (stratified squamous epithelium). The thickness of this lining varies with the menstrual cycle, and is thinner in the female child than in the mature woman.

> The thinness and immature structure of the vagina and external genitalia of children render these organs particularly susceptible to gonococcal infection. Gonococcal juvenile vaginitis is spread by contaminated bed-linen, towels, etc., and often occurs in children's institutions, where it may assume epidemic proportions. Female sex hormone is used in treating this condition, because it helps to make the mucous membrane temporarily thicker and also more resistant to this type of infection.

BREASTS

The mammary glands or breasts are closely connected with the reproductive system, and are under pituitary and sex hormone control. They are subject to marked changes at puberty, throughout pregnancy, during lactation, and after the menopause. The cyclic influence of the female hormones is demonstrated by the temporary breast swelling and soreness which often occur at each menstrual period.

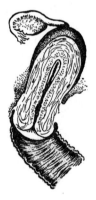

JUVENILE INTERNAL
GENITALIA

Male Reproductive System*

TESTES

The testes, or testicles, which lie in the abdomen during fetal life, pass downward through the inguinal canal and enter the scrotum shortly before birth.

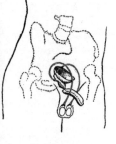

MALE REPRODUCTIVE SYSTEM
(AFTER G. W. CORNER)

> Failure of the testes to descend is known as cryptorchidism (G., *kryptos*, concealed + *orchis*, testicle). Sometimes, the process is merely delayed and takes place shortly after birth or during early childhood. If not, the testes may be brought to normal position by surgical operation, by endocrinologic treatment, or by both. Placement of the testes within the scrotum is important, because no spermatozoa will be produced while they remain within the abdomen.

The dual function of the testicle is the production of spermatozoa and the male sex hormone more or less constantly during the period of sexual maturity. The spermatozoa are produced within a series of slender canals, known as seminiferous tubules, which are imbedded in loose, connective tissue. This tissue contains the interstitial cells which secrete the male sex hormone.

EPIDIDYMES

The numerous seminiferous tubules come together into a smaller number of large tubes called efferent ducts, constituting an epididymis, attached to the testis. The secretion of the epididymis provides a suitable medium for the development of the spermatozoa during their passage through this structure.

VAS DEFERENTIA

The epididymis continues as the vas deferens which is a long tube extending from the scrotum through the inguinal

*See Plates V and VI.

canal into the abdominal cavity. It joins with the excretory duct of the seminal vesicle to form the ejaculatory duct, through which the semen passes during the orgasm. The ejaculatory duct from each side passes through the prostate and ends in the urethra.

SEMINAL VESICLES

The seminal vesicles are small club-shaped structures that produce a secretion necessary for the motility and transportation of the spermatozoa. It is also thought by some authorities (and denied by others) that the seminal vesicles act as reservoirs for the spermatozoa.

PROSTATE

The prostate gland is composed of muscular and glandular tissues and surrounds the upper portion of the urethra. It produces a secretion which facilitates and stimulates the motility of the spermatozoa. This secretion passes into the urethra through several small ducts.

PENIS

The penis is composed essentially of erectile tissue surrounding the urethra. The erectile tissue consists of blood spaces which, under the influence of sexual excitement, become distended with blood, thus rendering the organ erect.

During ejaculation, semen is deposited in the vagina. Semen contains spermatozoa and secretions of the epididymis, seminal vesicles, prostate and other glands. Normally, there are about 100 million spermatozoa per cubic centimeter of semen. These must be normally active in order to be able to penetrate the female genital system as far as the fallopian tubes. Although variations from the usual form occur in normal semen, a certain percentage of normal forms must be present for conception to take place.

The number, type and motility of the spermatozoa can be easily determined by microscopic examination. Certain terms are used to describe sperm disorders: azoospermia (G., *a*, without + *zoon*, animal + *sperma*, seed) means the absence of spermatozoa; oligospermia (G., *oligos*, few) indicates an insufficient number of spermatozoa; and necrospermia (G., *nekros*, dead) means that the spermatozoa are non-motile and therefore non-functioning; aspermia or aspermatism (G., *a*, without + *sperma*, seed) means lack of secretion or of expulsion of semen.

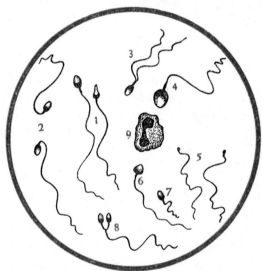

NORMAL AND ABNORMAL SPERMATOZOA

1 —normal (front and side view)	5 —pin head (microsperm)	8 —double head
2 —bent body	6 —tapering or pear-shaped head (pyriform)	9 —white blood cell (for comparison)
3 —double tail		
4 —giant head (megalosperm)	7 —short tail	

CHAPTER FIVE

CONTROL OF THE SEX HORMONES

Complete and normal development of the sexual organs and the secondary sex characteristics depend on the proper coordination of the gonads and the pituitary gland.

The anterior lobe of the pituitary gland secretes a number of hormones, among which are the gonadotropins (*gonad* + G., *tropos,* turning), which control the development and activity of the gonads. These, in turn, secrete the sex hormones essential for complete normal masculine or feminine development. The sex hormones, moreover, in certain amounts, have an inhibitory effect on the pituitary, suppressing or reducing the production of gonadotropins.

This reciprocal arrangement effects a delicate balance between the gonadotropic hormones and the various sex hormones, normally ensuring perfect control of sexual development and function. In brief, this basic concept of sex endocrinology is:

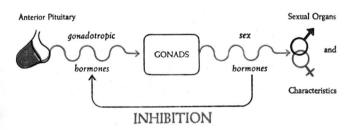

One of the gonadotropic hormones is known as the follicle-stimulating hormone. In the male it is responsible for the development of the tubules of the testes and the production of spermatozoa. In the female it is responsible for the cyclic stimulation of the ovarian follicle and ovulation. As the follicle develops, specialized cells within it produce the estrogenic hormone.

The other gonadotropic hormone produced by the anterior pituitary is the luteinizing hormone, which like the follicle-stimulating hormone acts upon the gonads of the male and female. In the male the luteinizing hormone stimulates the interstitial tissue within the testes to produce the male sex hormone. In the female the luteinizing hormone causes the development of specialized cells in the corpus luteum which in turn produce the corpus luteum hormone. The latter exerts its greatest influence in the second half of the menstrual cycle and during pregnancy.

It is thus apparent that for the maintenance of normal sexual development and function each gonadotropic hormone must be produced in proper quantity and at the proper time. Should the anterior pituitary fail in its task of production, not only will the gonads be affected adversely, but also, the secondary sex characteristics, which are dependent upon the hormone production of the gonads.

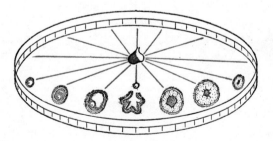

CHAPTER SIX

THE ESTROGENIC HORMONE

The estrogenic hormones are concerned not only with the stimulation of the sex urge in female animals and the preparation of the sexual organs for mating during estrus, but also with the general health and well-being of the body as a whole. In humans, where estrus as such does not exist, they play an important role in controlling body structure and in the development of genital organs and functions, including the menstrual cycle, particularly in its first half.

In addition to the true primary hormone, alpha-estradiol, found in animal ovaries, and the excretion products, estrone and estriol, obtained from placentae and urine, there is a group of lesser known estrogenic substances in plants, petroleum, coal and even in the waters and mud of the Dead Sea.

PHYSIOLOGY

In immature female animals, the administration of estrogens causes the precocious development of the sexual organs and the appearance of estrus. The uterus becomes enlarged and distended with a fluid secreted by the endometrium, and the vaginal epithelium becomes thickened and cornified. In addition, the mating reflexes develop and, under suitable conditions, the animal will receive the male.

These cornified vaginal layers desquamate in much the same manner as do the superficial cornified layers of the skin. If a loop or wire, or a pipette is introduced into the vagina and the content spread on a slide, stained, and examined microscopically, numerous large, cornified, non-nucleated cells will be seen. The presence of these cells represents the estrus phase of the sexual cycle. This vaginal smear test, usually performed on castrated female rats or mice, is used as a method of bio-assay of estrogenic preparations. According to Allen and Doisy who devised the test, a rat unit is the quantity of material necessary to produce a cornified vaginal smear in a castrate rat weighing 140 grams.

In humans, the estrogenic hormone plays a vital part not only in the reproductive function but also in the general well-being of woman. In addition to its role in the menstrual cycle, it has the following functions:

1. It maintains the normal size, capacity and functional activity of the accessory sex organs: uterus, fallopian tubes and vagina.

2. It preserves the normal epithelial layers of the vagina.

3. It influences normal uterine contractility by its stimulating effect on the muscular activity of the myometrium.

4. It promotes the growth of the duct tissue of the breast.

5. It acts upon the anterior pituitary so as to control the production of gonadotropic and other hormones.

6. It helps maintain the normal condition of the nasal and oral mucous membranes.

7. It is responsible for the womanliness of woman as expressed by the secondary sex characteristics: bodily contour, distribution of fat, distribution and growth of hair, breast development and psychic attitudes.

8. It has definite constitutional effects, directly reflected in the radiant physical and mental health of the normal, hormonally-balanced mature woman.

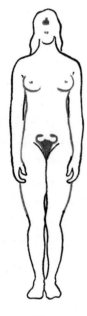

Tissues
INFLUENCED BY
ESTROGENS

THE MENSTRUAL CYCLE

Menstruation is a cyclic phenomenon occurring during the period of sexual maturity in woman, and represents a phase in the periodic preparation of the uterus to receive and nourish a fertilized ovum. It "marks a frustration of nature—the acknowledgment of failure of fertilization".

Normal cycles vary from 25 to 35 days; most commonly, the cycle is about 28 days and may be divided conveniently into three phases:

1. Proliferative, follicular or pre-ovulatory phase. This phase lasts about two weeks, counting from the first day of the previous menstruation. Under the influence of the follicle-stimulating hormone of the anterior pituitary, a graafian follicle containing an ovum matures, becomes distended with follicular fluid, and produces increasing amounts of follicular hormone. Stimulated by this latter hormone, the endometrium becomes thicker, and its glands develop and proliferate markedly. During this period of growth, the graafian follicle approaches the surface of the ovary and on the 12th to the 16th day, it ruptures and liberates the ovum. This is known as ovulation and marks the end of the proliferative phase. Subsequently, the ovum passes through the fallopian tube, and ultimately either leaves the uterus with the menstrual flow or, if fertilized, remains within it and develops into an embryo.

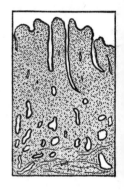

PROLIFERATIVE
ENDOMETRIUM

2. Secretory, progestational, luteal or post-ovulatory phase. This phase, which lasts about ten days, is characterized by the development of a new endocrine gland within the confines of the ruptured graafian follicle. A corpus luteum (L., *corpus*, body + *luteus*, yellow) forms, and secretes progesterone, the corpus luteum hormone, under the influence of the luteinizing hormone of the anterior

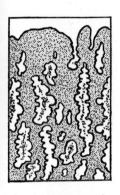

SECRETORY
ENDOMETRIUM

pituitary.* Now stimulated by progesterone, the endometrium becomes even more developed, its blood supply increases, and its glands actively secrete a mucoid material (secretory endometrium). Such an endometrium is able to receive and maintain a fertilized ovum; it is therefore, also called "progestational" (G., *pro*, in favor of + L., *gestatio*, from *gestare*, to bear).

3. Bleeding phase. If fertilization has not occurred, the corpus luteum regresses at about the 25th day. The resulting decrease in the corpus luteum hormone is considered responsible for the onset of menstruation several days later. The menses, which normally last about 4 days (range 3 to 6 days), mark the beginning of a new cycle. The menstrual fluid contains the sloughed off superficial layers of the endometrium, varying amounts of blood, and the unfertilized ovum. (Plate III)

> Menstruation usually presupposes ovulation. This is true in the majority of cases. However, it has been found that, occasionally, bleeding takes place without previous ovulation. This type of menstruation is often associated with anovulatory sterility and is termed pseudomenstruation or anovulatory menstruation. Other menstrual disorders are: dysmenorrhea (G., *dys*, difficult + *men*, month + *rhoia*, a flow)—painful menstruation; amenorrhea (G., *a*, without)—absence of menstruation; oligomenorrhea (G., *oligos*, little)—scanty or infrequent menstruation; meno-metrorrhagia (G., *men*, month + *metra*, uterus + *rhegnymi*, burst forth), also called functional uterine bleeding —excessive profuse bleeding from the uterus occurring at the menstrual period and also between periods, not due to organic causes.

*It is thus evident that, in contradistinction to the male gonad which, as far as we know, only secretes one hormone, testosterone, the female gonad secretes two, alpha-estradiol and progesterone. Not only menstruation, but also successful impregnation and maintenance of pregnancy depend on a suitable balance between these two hormones.

The menopause (L., *men*, month + *pausis*, cessation) is the permanent cessation of menstruation and is physiological when it occurs spontaneously during middle age. Artificial menopause occurs after the ovaries are removed or if induced by x-rays or radium. The climacteric (G., *klimakter*, the round of a ladder) is a particular epoch of later life when the body undergoes important aging changes. The female climacteric refers to the menopausal period. The male climacteric refers to the period of declining testicular function occurring in the latter middle age of men.

POTENCY AND UNITS

There exists much confusion today regarding the standardization of estrogenic products. A definite, crystalline compound like alpha-estradiol does not actually need bioassay, and its effects can be judged on the basis of weight alone. However, for the purposes of comparison with other estrogens, which are less pure or less active, alpha-estradiol is also assayed biologically in terms of Rat Units by the Allen-Doisy method.

The Rat Unit (R.U.) is the biological assay unit developed by Allen and Doisy, and is applicable to all estrogenic substances, in contrast to the International Unit (I.U.) referring only to estrone. The comparative potency of the three naturally occurring estrogens on the basis of hormone weight is as follows:

> 1 mg. of alpha-estradiol   ⇌   12,000 R.U.
> 1 mg. of estrone (theelin) ⇌   1,000 R.U.
> 1 mg. of estriol (theelol)   ⇌   150 R.U.

It is thus seen that alpha-estradiol is 12 times as potent as estrone and 80 times as potent as estriol.

At a time when estrone was widely used, the International Unit was devised. This was arbitrarily defined as the effect

37

of 0.0001 mg. (or 0.1 gamma*) of an average sample of various estrone preparations.

The relationship between the two units can be determined from the following equations:

1 mg. estrone $\rightleftharpoons$ 10,000 I.U. (so defined)
1 mg. estrone $\rightleftharpoons$ 1,000 R.U. (by actual bio-assay)
Therefore, 1 R.U. $\rightleftharpoons$ 10 I.U.

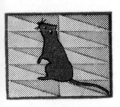

ONE RAT UNIT

ONE
INTERNATIONAL
UNIT

With this ratio in mind, the comparative activity of the estrogenic hormones may be expressed in terms of both units:

1 mg. alpha-estradiol $\rightleftharpoons$ 12,000 R.U. or 120,000 I.U.
1 mg. estrone (theelin) $\rightleftharpoons$ 1,000 R.U. or 10,000 I.U.
1 mg. estriol (theelol) $\rightleftharpoons$ 150 R.U. or 1,500 I.U.

From this table, it is evident that a much smaller quantity of alpha-estradiol is required to accomplish the same therapeutic effect in a given patient. It is this fact which explains the striking economy and efficiency of alpha-estradiol preparations.

ESTROGENIC HORMONE PREPARATIONS

Alpha-estradiol, the primary estrogenic hormone, is available as the free hormone and in its esterified forms, the benzoate and the dipropionate.

Alpha-estradiol, dihydrotheelin, the follicular hormone, is supplied in tablets and solution for oral use, and in ointment, suppositories and nasal spray for local use, under the name of PROGYNON-DH.

The benzoate of estradiol, the most highly effective ester with prolonged action, in ampules for intramuscular injec-

*One gamma (γ) is equivalent to 0.001 mg.

tion, is PROGYNON-B.

The *di*propionate of estradiol, for even more prolonged action (though of lower potency), in ampules for injection, is PROGYNON-DP.

The definite advantages of these preparations are of practical interest. They contain the various forms of the primary estrogenic hormone in exactly known quantity, in chemically pure, crystalline form, stable to changes in climate, uninfluenced by storage, naturally well tolerated in the body, and of surpassing therapeutic potency. These preparations, adapted to various modes of administration, represent a truly versatile method of estrogenic therapy. Since they contain the most potent estrogenic hormone known, a distinct economy is achieved, both as to quantity of hormone which need be administered and as to the cost of treatment.

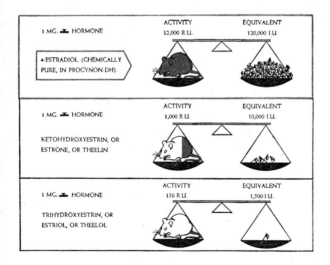

CHAPTER SEVEN

ESTROGENIC HORMONE THERAPY

The follicular hormone is employed therapeutically on the basis of certain of its physiological actions. In general, estrogen therapy utilizes the following effects of the hormone:

1. *Developmental action on the reproductive organs.* In hypogonadism (also called hypogenitalism or sexual infantilism), estrogens are administered in order to obtain developmental effects (e.g., growth of the uterus and breasts) not yet attained because of the insufficient supply of the patient's own estrogenic hormone. This is called replacement therapy.

2. *Inhibition of pituitary hormones.* This action is utilized in controlling excessive or unwanted lactation (milk secretion) after delivery,* and in the treatment of the menopausal syndrome, where estrogen therapy makes possible a smooth and comfortable transition to the new state of lowered ovarian activity.

3. *Constitutional effects* in both younger and older women where the estrogenic hormone produces an increase in muscle strength, bodily vigor, and mental faculties. These

---

*Lactation is under the influence of the lactogenic (L., *lac*, milk + G., *gennao*, produce) hormone of the anterior pituitary, also called prolactin (G., *pro*, in favor of + L., *lac*, milk). This hormone is used as a galactogogue (G., *galakt*, milk + *agogos*, leading) when milk production is inadequate. Its secretion by the pituitary is depressed by adequate amounts of estrogenic hormone. Thus, stimulation and suppression of milk secretion after delivery is now possible by endocrinologic methods.

effects are consistently present during the administration of the follicular hormone for other purposes, e.g., treatment of the menopausal syndrome, and constitute an important factor in the patient's restoration to full health. Beneficial constitutional effects are notably absent during treatment with the unnatural artificial estrogens, such as stilbestrol.

PRINCIPAL CLINICAL INDICATIONS

The Menopausal Syndrome

The menopause is truly "a change of life", not only in regard to the cessation of menstruation, but also because the many symptoms and disturbances that so frequently accompany it produce such profound changes in physical and mental health that the patient's activity and usefulness as a member of society may be materially curtailed.

SYMPTOMS

The train of symptoms included in the menopausal syndrome are alternating hot flushes and sweats, dizziness, headache, palpitation, numbness, tingling and insomnia. In addition, there may be emotional and nervous disturbances, such as irritability, excitability, nervousness, impairment of memory, failure of concentration, easy fatigability, neurasthenia and depression. Occasionally, actual psychosis may develop. The most important psychotic manifestation at the menopause is involutional melancholia, characterized by a state of profound depression and altered contact with reality. Although the mode of action is not yet entirely known, estrogen therapy has been reported to be frequently of benefit.

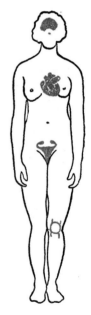

Organs
INVOLVED IN
MENOPAUSAL
SYNDROME

41

The widest use of the follicular hormone is in the treatment of the menopausal syndrome. Usually, at the outset of treatment, the required amount (in divided doses injected two or three times a week) is about 20,000 R.U. weekly in the most severe cases; 12,000 R.U. weekly in the moderately severe cases; and 4,000 R.U. or less in the milder types. This dosage may be administered for one month or longer, until the symptoms are controlled, and then is gradually reduced to a level that will keep the patient comfortable (maintenance level). Eventually, after the transitional period has been passed, it may be possible to stop estrogen therapy completely.

The follicular hormone may be given by injection (PROGYNON-B or PROGYNON-DP Ampules), or by mouth (PROGYNON-DH Tablets or Solution), or both. Oral therapy (one PROGYNON-DH Tablet of 0.5 mg. two or three times daily, or 10 to 20 drops of PROGYNON-DH Solution twice daily) is particularly useful in mild cases or as maintenance therapy of controlled severe cases, where it may constitute complete therapy. In general, these oral forms are valuable whenever the patient cannot be seen sufficiently often by the physician. Periodic observation is necessary, nevertheless, in order to avoid self medication and unwarranted dependence on estrogens. Likewise, examination at regular intervals permits adjustment of dosage and diminishes the possibility of the patient neglecting herself.

Progress in treatment may be judged by the diminution in number or disappearance of the flushes and sweats, by the relief of irritability, insomnia and fatigue, and by the general improvement in the well-being of the patient. An objective method of determining the response to estrogen therapy is by studying the vaginal smear or spread.

Estrogen therapy, administered for relief of the menopausal symptoms is reflected by a measurable degree of cornification of the vaginal epithelium. The required dose for full cornification (full dosage) may be termed a "human unit", which, for many patients, is equivalent to 2,000 to 3,000 R.U. daily, although marked individual variations occur.

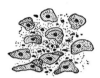

atrophic

OTHER MENOPAUSAL DISTURBANCES

Other disturbances which occasionally occur at the menopause are amenable to estrogen therapy, e.g., menopausal arthritis and menopausal hypertension. Dosage for menopausal arthralgia is usually 10,000 R.U. PROGYNON-B administered at the outset, two to three times weekly; while dosage for hypertension associated with the menopause is to be judged by the underlying estrogen deficiency.

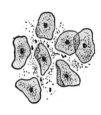

moderate estrogen deficiency

Senile atrophy of the vagina and external genitalia, associated with itching and usually postmenopausal, is a result of declining ovarian function, and as such responds to estrogen injection therapy, especially when it is combined with local treatment in the form of vaginal suppositories or ointment containing the free hormone (PROGYNON-DH Suppositories and Ointment).

Dosage consists of vulvar inunctions of 2 grams per day of PROGYNON-DH Ointment containing 1800 R.U. per gram, reduced, with improvement, to ointment containing 360 R.U. per gram. In senile vaginitis, one PROGYNON-DH Suppository of 4800 R.U. is inserted nightly, dosage being reduced with improvement to suppositories of 480 R.U. Concomitant systemic therapy may be given as 6000 R.U. of PROGYNON-B two to three times weekly.

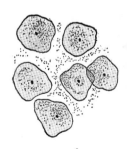

normal

TYPES OF VAGINAL
SMEARS

The Hypo-ovarian State

Incomplete sexual development, variously referred to as hypogonadism, hypogenitalism, sexual infantilism, sexual juvenilism, etc., usually is the result of a deficiency of ovarian activity. (Plate IV)

SYMPTOMS

This hypo-ovarian state, which may be manifested by a variety of symptoms including amenorrhea or oligomenorrhea, dysmenorrhea, sterility, frigidity and underdeveloped breasts, is associated with underdevelopment of the sex organs.

TREATMENT

The treatment of these symptoms is essentially the treatment of the underlying hypo-ovarian state. Therapy may be (1) *substitutive* or *replacement*, furnishing the estrogenic hormone in cyclic dosage with the object of producing sufficient development of the secondary sex organs, so that ultimately they may function adequately under the effect of the patient's own hormone; or (2) *stimulative*, consisting of an effort to stimulate the patient's own ovaries to normal cyclic activity by means of the gonadotropic hormones contained in pregnant mare serum (ANTERON*), after the accessory sex organs have been previously developed with estrogen therapy.

Treatment usually consists of follicular hormone for a period of two weeks; the hormone is then discontinued for two weeks; and then treatment is resumed—producing thus a series of hormone cycles for at least several months.

*See page 81.

PROGYNON-B, (6,000 to 10,000 R.U.) may be given three times weekly, by intramuscular injection, for two weeks, supplemented on alternate days by two to four 0.5 mg. tablets of PROGYNON-DH.

To produce complete hormonal cycles more closely approximating the normal events of the menstrual cycle, corpus luteum hormone (PROLUTON) is given during the intervals between follicular hormone therapy.

Amenorrhea

Amenorrhea, most obvious manifestation of the hypo-ovarian state, is the result of follicular hormone deficiency, usually reflected in subnormal development of the sex organs and the secondary sex characteristics. It is customarily divided into two types: (1) primary amenorrhea, i.e., menstruation has never occurred in a patient well beyond the age of puberty; and (2) secondary amenorrhea, i.e., cessation of menstruation which had occurred previously for a variable time. Both express, in general, a profound estrogenic deficiency which may be especially severe in older patients with the primary type. Treatment of both types is essentially as described for the hypo-ovarian state. Secondary amenorrhea usually responds more readily, however.

As a result of estrogen therapy, the amenorrheic patient has the psychological satisfaction of menstruating regularly, of "being like other women". In addition, there is progressive development of the sex organs and secondary sex characteristics so that, after several months of treatment, some patients will have normal, spontaneous menstrual cycles. Others may require supplementary gonad-stimulating therapy with pregnant mare serum hormone (ANTERON*) in

*See page 81.

order to "pick up the rhythm" that has been established. Occasionally, thyroid therapy is required in certain cases.

Dysmenorrhea

Dysmenorrhea, "painful periods" or "uterine cramps", may be due to organic causes, such as uterine fibroids or pelvic inflammation, or may be functional, i.e., without previous disease or demonstrable deformity.

Functional dysmenorrhea, with which we are here concerned, is generally associated with hormonal imbalance of two main types:

(1) Estrogenic deficiency and uterine underdevelopment, amenable to treatment with the follicular hormone (PROGYNON). This is the rarer type. Dosage is usually 6000 R.U. PROGYNON-B two or three times weekly by injection during the first two weeks of the cycle; the course is repeated for several months.

(2) Normal sexual development but with unusually contractile or overactive uterus. This is the more frequent type. The excessive uterine contractions result from stimulation of the uterine muscle by the *hormone of the posterior lobe* of the pituitary, uncontrolled because of insufficient secretion of corpus luteum hormone,* which may be replaced with PRANONE Tablets by mouth or PROLUTON by injection.

Sterility

Sterility may be due to either the male or female partner, or both. Infertile women may be divided into three groups: (1) Those with symptoms of hypogonadism are best treated for that condition, using female sex hormone for its developmental actions. (2) Those with no impairment of sexual development are suitable for gonad-stimulating therapy

*See page 57.

with gonadotropic hormone of pregnant mare serum, in order to stimulate the ovary to maturation and liberation of the ova. (3) Those with organic disease, such as uterine fibroids or inflammation of the neck of the uterus or of the fallopian tubes, are not endocrine problems as such, and are best treated with other measures.

The dosage of PROGYNON for the treatment of sterility in hypogonadal women is that required for the treatment of the hypo-ovarian state.

Frigidity

Frigidity (L., *frigidus,* cold) or sexual coldness in women is an extremely prevalent and difficult problem. Although often of psychic origin, e.g., domestic incompatibility, it may also be one feature of estrogenic deficiency along with underdeveloped genital organs, irregular or scanty menstruation, immature sexual attitude, etc., and, as such, may be amenable to correction by the administration of follicular hormone.

The effects of successful estrogen therapy in hypogonadal young women include:

1. The growth of the external and internal genitalia and the onset of menstruation, and the development of the secondary sex characteristics, including the breasts and the axillary and pubic hair.

2. A moderate increase in body weight, most noticeable in the buttocks, thighs, and hips, producing a characteristic feminine appearance.

3. An increase in muscle strength, bodily vigor and mental acumen.

4. An increase in sex consciousness with a corresponding change in emotional status. The use of cosmetics, in-

creased attention to the details of dress and normal interest in the opposite sex are external manifestations of this important change.

Underdeveloped Breasts

Abnormally small breasts may occur with other symptoms of hypogonadism, or as an isolated symptom. In either case, the breasts may be developed by estrogen therapy, particularly when supplemented by local inunction treatment. It has been shown that estrogens can be absorbed through the skin of the human female into the breast tissue, and by this route can produce their characteristic stimulation of mammary growth. (Plate IV)

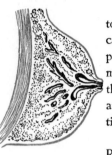

PROGYNON-DH may be administered in doses of 12,000 R.U., or more, weekly (daily inunction of ointment containing 1800 R.U. per gram—one gram per day), or 360 R.U. per gram (five grams daily). The daily dose is divided in two equal portions for inunction over each breast. Supplementary injections of PROGYNON-B (6,000 R.U. two or three times weekly) are of value, particularly when other symptoms of hypogonadism are present.

Juvenile Vaginitis

Gonorrheal vulvovaginitis of children or juvenile vaginitis may be successfully treated by temporarily converting the thin, immature juvenile vaginal epithelium into a more resistant type. This treatment, which is harmless and widely employed, consists of inserting, nightly, one juvenile vaginal suppository containing 480 R.U. of PROGYNON-DH, for a period of three to eight weeks as determined by weekly smear examinations for gonococci. Oral therapy in equivalent dosage is often employed, using one 0.5 mg. PROGYNON-DH Tablet daily, and upwards.

Sagittal section of female pelvic anatomy

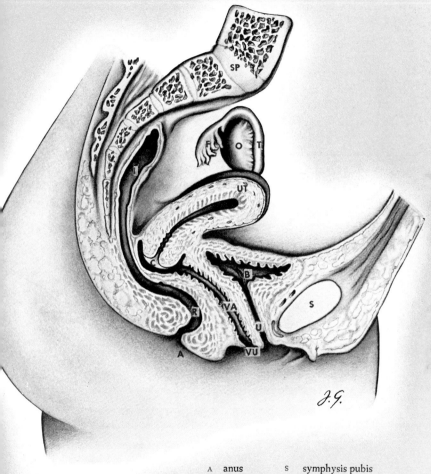

J.G.

A	anus	S	symphysis pubis
B	bladder	SP	spine
C	cervix	T	fallopian tube
F	fimbria	U	urethra
I	intestine	UT	uterus
O	ovary	VA	vagina
R	rectum	VU	vulva

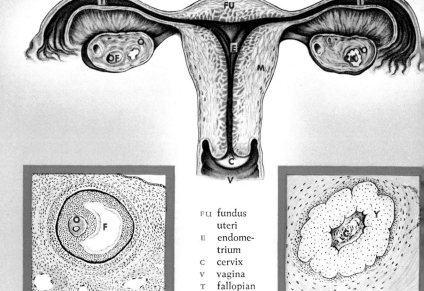

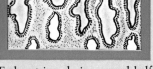

Mature ovarian follicle showing
ovum (o) and follicular fluid (f)

FU fundus
    uteri
E   endome-
    trium
C   cervix
V   vagina
T   fallopian
    tube
O   ovary
OF ovarian
    follicle
CL corpus
    luteum
M   myome-
    trium

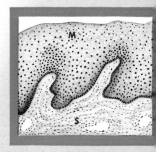

Mature corpus luteum showin
yellow body (y) and blood clot (

Endometrium during second half
of menstrual cycle

Vaginal epithelium showing m
cosa (m) and submucosa (s)

PLATE II

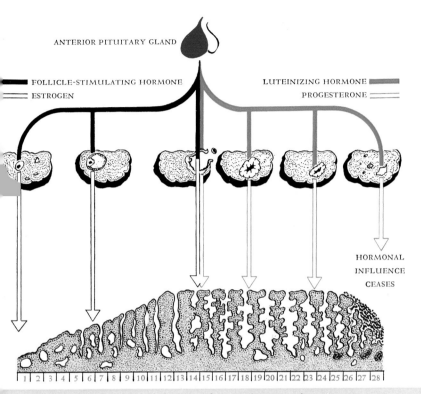

Diagrammatic Representation of the Influence of Hormones on the Ovary and Endometrium

The anterior pituitary gland secretes the gonadotropic hormones which stimulate the ovary, viz., the follicle-stimulating hormone and the luteinizing hormone. The follicle-stimulating hormone, as its name implies, stimulates an immature ovarian follicle to grow, an action which takes place during the first half of the menstrual cycle. During the process of growth, the ovum contained within the follicle matures, and the estrogenic hormone, alpha-estradiol, is secreted by the ovarian follicular epithelium. Estrogen causes the endo-metrial glandular tissue to proliferate. Following ovulation in the middle of the menstrual cycle, the corpus luteum forms from the ovarian follicle. The corpus luteum is stimulated by the luteinizing hormone to secrete progesterone. Progesterone, in turn, adds its influ-ence to the endometrium causing the latter structure to enter upon the secretory phase during the second half of the menstrual cycle. (Actually, secretory or progestational endometrium results from the influence of both progesterone and estrogen, but for the sake of simplicity, graphic representation of the action of estrogen in the latter half of the cycle has been omitted.) About the twenty-sixth day of the cycle, the influence of both progesterone and alpha-estradiol is suddenly withdrawn. The endometrium undergoes degeneration followed by menstruation.

PLATE III

Twenty year old hypogonad female with primary amenorrhea

COURTESY RITA S. FINKLER, M.D.

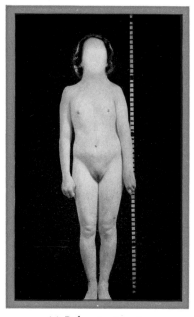
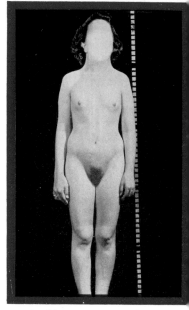

(a) Before treatment   (b) After one year's treatment

Breast growth produced by PROGYNON-DH Ointment

COURTESY CYRIL M. MACBRYDE, M.D.

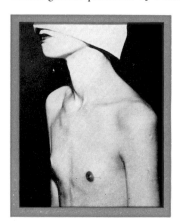
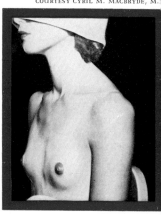

(a) Before treatment   (b) After two months' treatment

PLATE IV

Sagittal section of male genitalia

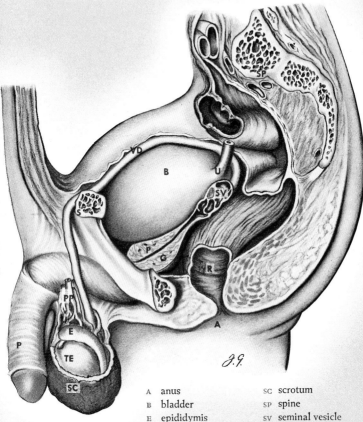

A	anus	SC	scrotum
B	bladder	SP	spine
E	epididymis	SV	seminal vesicle
PG	prostate gland	TE	testis
P	penis	U	ureter
R	rectum	VD	vas deferens
S	symphysis pubis	PP	pampiniform plexus

PLATE V

Microscopic section of seminiferous tubules (AFTER MAXIMOW)

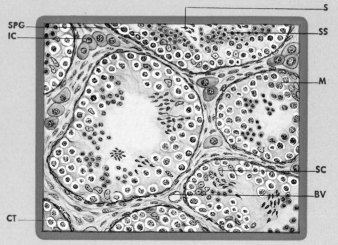

SPG spermatogonium	S sperm	SC Sertoli cells
IC interstitial cells	SS secondary spermatocytes	BV blood vessel
CT connective tissue cells	M mitoses of spermatocytes	

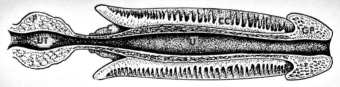

Cross-section of penis

P prostate gland	C Cowper's gland	CC corpus cavernosum
UT utricle	U urethra	GP glans penis

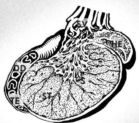

Cross-section of testicle

DD ductus deferens	SV spermatic veins	S septum
TE tail of epididymis	ST seminiferous tubules	HE head of epididymis

PLATE VI

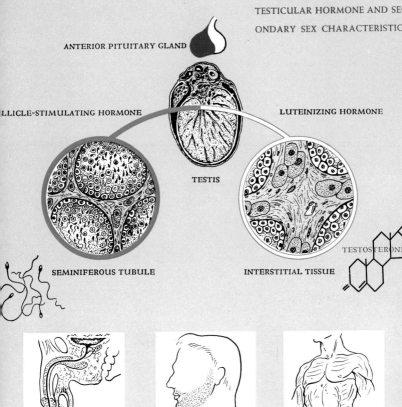

ANTERIOR PITUITARY GLAND

FOLLICLE-STIMULATING HORMONE

LUTEINIZING HORMONE

TESTIS

SEMINIFEROUS TUBULE

INTERSTITIAL TISSUE

TESTOSTERONE

Under the influence of the anterior pituitary hormone, the testes mature and develop as follows: The *follicle-stimulating gonadotropic hormone* (FSH) initiates and maintains spermatogenesis within the seminiferous tubules. The *luteinizing hormone* (LH) stimulates the interstitium of the testes to secrete the male sex hormone, testosterone. Testosterone, in turn, exerts profound and wide-spread effects in the male, being responsible for the development of adult genitalia and secondary sex characteristics, such as distribution of hair and greater muscular development.

PLATE VII

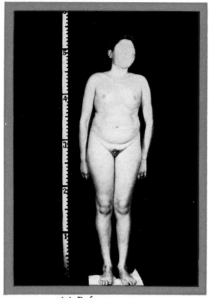 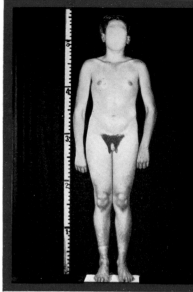

(a) Before treatment   (b) After treatment

Sixteen and one-half year old eunuchoid male whose testes had never descende
ORETON-M Tablets were administered over a six months' period. Note masculin
zation of body configuration, loss of girdle fat, and growth of genitalia.

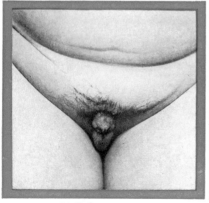 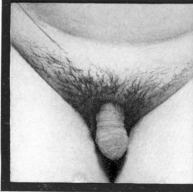

(a) Before treatment   (b) After treatment

Genital development following 3½ months' treatment COURTESY JOSEPH EIDELSBERG, M.

PLATE VIII

Suppression of Lactation

When it is desired to suppress the flow of milk in the breast, as upon the miscarriage, death or illness of the child, or if maternal illness supervenes, or in ordinary weaning, large doses of follicular hormone are found effective: 10,000 R.U. of PROGYNON-B may be administered twice daily for two days.

The action depends on the suppression by estrogenic hormone of the pituitary lactogenic hormone (or prolactin). Since the latter usually begins to act about the third day after delivery, treatment is best begun at that time. Similar prolactin inhibition may be achieved with male sex hormone therapy which is preferred by most clinicians.

Other Indications

In addition to the well-established indications for estrogen therapy described above, there are others where estrogens are employed more or less empirically or experimentally.

NAUSEA AND VOMITING OF PREGNANCY

Estrogenic deficiency has been reported in some cases of nausea and vomiting of pregnancy, and small doses of follicular hormone have been administered to overcome the condition.

If the patient can tolerate medication by mouth, 0.2 mg. tablets of PROGYNON-DH may be given daily; if not, 500 R.U. of PROGYNON-B may be injected every second day until vomiting ceases.

MIGRAINE

Migraine, which is a symptom rather than a disease, has many causes, one of which may be estrogenic insufficiency.

A patient in whom there is a consistent relation between the menstrual cycle and the time of onset of recurring attacks of migraine merits a trial of estrogen therapy. Paradoxically, follicular hormone therapy has been found successful not only in women, but also in men subject to migraine.

A therapeutic test consists of 6000 to 10,000 R.U. every second day for three to four weeks, so planned that treatment is well under way to prevent an anticipated attack.

NEUROSES AND PSYCHONEUROSES

The most characteristic neurotic and psychotic disorders associated with estrogenic insufficiency are those occurring at the menopause. However, since deficiency of the follicular hormone may occur in other age groups, it is important to consider this factor in the evaluation of nervous and mental disorders of women. A course of full replacement therapy as described under the hypo-ovarian state of the menopause will generally suffice to indicate whether ovarian deficiency is a contributory or causative factor.

ATROPHIC RHINITIS

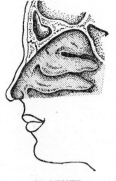

AREA INVOLVED
IN ATROPHIC
RHINITIS

Atrophic rhinitis, or ozena (G., *ozaina,* stench) is a chronic disease of the nose of unknown origin, characterized by marked thinning of the mucous membrane, decrease in size of the internal bones of the nose, crust-formation, and the production of an extremely foul odor.

On the basis of an evolutionary sexual relation among various tissues of the body, and experimental observations, estrogens have been employed in the treatment of this disease with favorable results. PROGYNON-DH Nasal Spray has been prepared especially for use in this condition.

CHAPTER EIGHT

THE CORPUS LUTEUM HORMONE

Reproduction—from the stage of fertilization to the birth of a living child—is dependent upon endocrine factors. The hormone most directly concerned with the preparation for, and the maintenance of pregnancy, is the corpus luteum hormone, found both in the corpus luteum and placenta, and obtainable in pure crystalline form.

PHYSIOLOGY

The corpus luteum hormone is responsible for the secretory or progestational phase of the menstrual cycle, which represents a periodic preparation of the endometrium for the reception and nourishment of a fertilized ovum. If fertilization does not take place, the corpus luteum regresses and menstruation occurs.

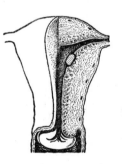

COMMON SITE OF IMPLANTATION OF FERTILIZED OVUM

If the uterus of an immature rabbit is prepared by previous injections of estrogen, progesterone will cause a typical progestational endometrium. This was used as a quantitative test by Clauberg, who used immature rabbits which first received ten injections of estrogen, then a 5 day course of progesterone.

A similar test is the Corner-Allen test, performed on adult rabbits which are first mated, then castrated. A Corner-Allen Rabbit Unit is the amount of corpus luteum hormone which, divided into five daily doses, produces, by the sixth day, a condition of the uterus equal to that on the eighth day of a normal pregnancy.

When fertilization of the ovum takes place, the fertilized ovum passes from the fallopian tube into the uterus where it implants itself into the progestational endometrium that has been prepared for it. After nidation, the embryo develops, along with the placenta and other structures.

The developing ovum, which becomes the embryo, is surrounded by a set of structures that have to do with its vital functions: nutrition, respiration, elimination and protection.

Immediately surrounding the embryo is a sac-like structure, the amnion, containing clear watery fluid, the amniotic fluid. This bag of waters, serves as a protective watery cushion. At the time of birth, it forms a fluid wedge to help dilate the cervix of the uterus.

Outside the amnion is the chorion, part of which is attached to the uterine wall by means of delicate projections called villi. Its main function is nutrition. These organs are known as the fetal membranes.

The placenta consists of a portion of the endometrium which has become highly developed and filled with blood vessels, connected with a similarly developed part of the chorion. The umbilical cord containing blood vessels is attached to this region. Maternal and fetal blood are in contact in the placenta which thus serves as the connecting link between mother and embryo. In addition to these vital functions, certain cells of the placenta produce progesterone, estrogens and gonadotropic hormones.

After conception, the corpus luteum hormone is first secreted by the corpus luteum, which, instead of regressing, as does the corpus luteum of menstruation, becomes larger and secretes its hormone in increasing amounts.

About the third or fourth month of pregnancy, the pla-

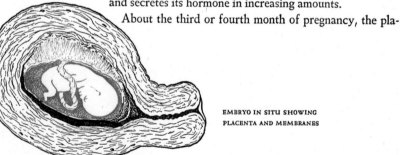

EMBRYO IN SITU SHOWING
PLACENTA AND MEMBRANES

centa takes over the function of secreting progesterone. This period of transition from the corpus luteum to the placenta is a critical stage of early pregnancy; and a deficiency of a hormone at this time may result in abortion.

> The duration of normal pregnancy is approximately nine months in the human female: this is called full term pregnancy. If the fetus is expelled during the first three months of the pregnancy, the process is called abortion. (In the lay sense, abortion is generally associated with criminal or induced abortion. According to medical usage, abortion, unless otherwise specified, refers to early termination of pregnancy due to any cause whatever.)
>
> If the fetus is expelled during the fourth, fifth or sixth month, the process is called miscarriage. Some authorities do not differentiate between abortion and miscarriage, and use the terms synonymously. Premature labor is birth between the sixth and ninth month.
>
> Certain women abort repeatedly during successive pregnancies, usually about the third month. This is called habitual abortion. Occasionally, a pregnant woman may have uterine cramps and bleeding, due to threatened abortion.

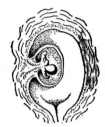

4-6 WEEKS

As pregnancy progresses, various hormonal and other changes take place preparatory to labor. The mechanism of labor is exceedingly complex, and as yet is not completely understood. However, it is fairly certain that two of the most important factors causing onset of labor are: (1) a decrease in the production of corpus luteum hormone just prior to labor, and (2) the increasing sensitivity of the uterine muscle to the oxytocic action of the posterior pituitary hormone. It has been shown that these factors are directly connected, and that corpus luteum hormone aids in reducing uterine contractility.

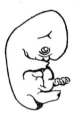

12-16 WEEKS

In habitual abortion regularly taking place during the early stages of pregnancy, marked deficiency of corpus luteum hormone has been reported frequently. If the hor-

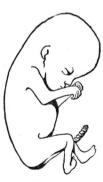

53

5-7 MONTHS

mone level is kept up to normal by the administration of large doses of PROLUTON (pure corpus luteum hormone) abortion may be prevented and pregnancy may go on to full term.

Corpus luteum hormone aids in breast development—it acts on the acinar or glandular portion of the breast, while the follicular hormone, as noted previously, promotes the growth of the duct tissue.

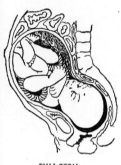

FULL TERM
PREGNANCY

POTENCY AND UNITS

Since corpus luteum hormone is available in pure crystalline form of unvarying potency and composition, dosage is expressed in milligrams. One International Unit is equivalent to one milligram.*

CORPUS LUTEUM PREPARATIONS

The corpus luteum hormone, progesterone, is available as PROLUTON, in ampules for injection.

The orally effective progestin, anhydrohydroxy-progesterone, is available as PRANONE, in tablets for oral use. Approximately five milligrams of PRANONE have the clinical effect, when given orally, of one milligram of PROLUTON by injection. All the clinical effects of PROLUTON therapy are achieved with PRANONE by mouth. These preparations represent the only efficient method of progestin therapy. "Ovarian pills" or "corpus luteum pills" have absolutely no hormonal action and no place in modern endocrinologic therapy.

---

*Biological units for progesterone, such as rabbit units, are now obsolete. However, the following equivalents may be noted for completeness. 1 mg. progesterone ⇌ 1 Corner-Allen Rabbit Unit ⇌ 1.3 to 2 Clauberg Units ⇌ 1 International Unit.

CHAPTER NINE

CORPUS LUTEUM HORMONE THERAPY

Corpus luteum hormone therapy is based on the following physiological effects.

1. Production of secretory endometrium. As shown in the previous chapter, normal menstruation is preceded by a secretory or progestational phase, under the influence of the corpus luteum hormone. A large proportion of cases of meno-metrorrhagia or functional uterine bleeding show an arrest of the endometrial cycle in the proliferative phase without the normal progression to the secretory phase. This is usually due to corpus luteum deficiency, and may be corrected by administration of PROLUTON.

2. Inhibition of uterine motility. The inhibitory effect of PROLUTON on the contractility of the uterus is of importance not only in the protection of pregnancy, but also in relation to dysmenorrhea. One or two days before the onset of menstruation, there is a rapid decline in corpus luteum hormone and removal of its restraining effect on uterine motility, which, in some women, causes dysmenorrhea. Such dysmenorrhea may be relieved by supplying the deficient hormone by mouth as PRANONE, or by injection as PROLUTON.

3. Metabolism of estrogens. Both hormones produced by the ovary are in a state of constant balance in the normal female. A factor in the maintenance of this balance is the

metabolic effect of progesterone on alpha-estradiol resulting in the urinary end-products, estrone and estriol. This effect is utilized in the relief of premenstrual tension with corpus luteum hormone, since there is an excessive amount of circulating estrogen in this disorder.

PRINCIPAL CLINICAL INDICATIONS

Habitual Abortion

A pregnant woman with a history of previous spontaneous abortion requires scrupulous supervision by her physician. In addition to the customary practice of avoiding strenuous exercise, excessive fatigue, highly emotional states, long automobile rides, and sexual intercourse during the first three months, PROLUTON therapy is indicated, particularly between the tenth and sixteenth weeks, the time of greatest hazard. Many clinicians administer PROLUTON or PRANONE to patients with a history of habitual abortion as soon as the diagnosis of pregnancy is established.

Corpus luteum hormone is given either by injection as 2 to 5 mg. PROLUTON three times weekly, or by mouth as two 5 mg. tablets of PRANONE daily, as the basic dosage. When the patient is subjected to unusual physical or emotional stress, dosage is increased to 5 mg. PROLUTON by daily injection, or two to three 10 mg. PRANONE Tablets daily.

Threatened Abortion

When a pregnant woman shows signs of threatened abortion, such as uterine cramps or vaginal bleeding, she requires immediate and energetic treatment, irrespective of previous pregnancies or abortions. The usual measures of bed rest and sedatives are supplemented by adequate doses of PROLUTON. As long as pain or bleeding is present, 10 mg. of PROLUTON are injected daily, reducing to 5 mg. daily when the symptoms have subsided.

Dysmenorrhea

Functional dysmenorrhea due to a deficiency or imbalance in corpus luteum hormone at the time of menstruation may be effectively treated with the hormone either by injection or by mouth. For this purpose, PRANONE Tablets 5 or 10 mg. may be given once or twice daily for the last eight to ten days preceding menstruation; alternatively, PROLUTON 1 to 2 mg. daily (up to 5 mg.) may be administered during the same period of time.

Corpus luteum hormone therapy corrects an underlying disturbance in a physiologic manner, in contrast to various anodyne or analgesic preparations, which are merely directed at the symptoms.

In addition to relieving dysmenorrhea,* administration of the hormone often results in the relief of other troublesome menstrual symptoms, such as headaches and breast pains. Moreover, freedom from painful periods frequently persists even after therapy is stopped.

Corpus luteum hormone therapy does not interfere with the endometrial cycle, ovulation, or fertility. On the contrary, it has been noted that a considerable number of infertile women who were receiving PROLUTON for dysmenorrhea became pregnant for the first time, as though relative corpus luteum deficiency had been the cause of their sterility as well as their dysmenorrhea.

*In the especially difficult and refractory cases, not responding to usual methods of treatment, male sex hormone may be administered (see page 72).

Premenstrual Tension

In some women, menstruation is preceded by a state of nervous and physical tension, which may often be extremely disagreeable and troublesome. This is called premenstrual tension, and is characterized by fatigue, irritability, headache, backache, insomnia, unreasonable emotional outbursts, extreme annoyance with trifles and a foreboding sensation of indescribable tension, as if the patient "would like to jump out of her skin".

This condition is ascribed to excessive amounts of estrogen in the blood during the three or four days preceding the menses. Since corpus luteum hormone is concerned in the metabolism and elimination of estrogen, the administration of PROLUTON and PRANONE frequently results in marked relief from the tension. Dosage is the same as in the treatment of functional dysmenorrhea.

Functional Uterine Bleeding

Excessive or unduly prolonged uterine bleeding at menstrual periods and/or during the intermenstrual periods is often characterized by the persistence of a proliferative type of uterine endometrium (an arrest in the first phase of the cycle). The lack of the normal progression to the secretory phase is due to a deficiency of corpus luteum hormone. PROLUTON may be administered in order to correct the situation.

During the ten days before the patient is expected to menstruate, 2 mg. PROLUTON may be injected daily, or 5 mg. on alternate days. The oral equivalent is 10 to 20 mg. PRANONE daily, in divided doses.

However, when hypogonadism or depressed ovarian function is present in addition to the bleeding, it is advisable to prepare the endometrium and render it more receptive by first administering the follicular hormone. This is full cycle therapy and consists of 6000 R.U. of PROGYNON-B twice weekly, or three 0.5 mg. PROGYNON-DH Tablets daily during the first half of the cycle, followed by PROLUTON or PRANONE in the dosage described above during the second half of the cycle. In this way, the effects of the normally functioning ovary upon the endometrium may be completely restored.

After several cycles of replacement therapy with corpus luteum hormone alone or combined with estrogen, some investigators recommend stimulative therapy with gonadotropic hormones of pregnant mare serum in order to stimulate the ovary to normal function.

When bleeding is unusually profuse and persistent, it may be checked by administering male sex hormone* in adequate doses. After establishing control of the bleeding, substitutive therapy with PROLUTON in the second half of the cycle, or stimulative therapy with ANTERON (pregnant mare serum hormone) in the first half of the cycle may be instituted.†

Toxemia of Pregnancy

The high blood pressure and other features of pregnancy toxemia are believed by some investigators to be due to an imbalance between follicular hormone and corpus luteum hormone, probably comprising a relative deficiency of the latter. The administration of corpus luteum hormone to toxemic patients has resulted in a decrease in the number of maternal and fetal deaths. The use of the hormone in this condition is still experimental.

*See page 72.
†See page 81.

CHAPTER TEN

THE MALE SEX HORMONE

Because of their masculinizing properties, androgens, particularly testosterone, the male sex hormone, are capable of preventing castration changes and of inducing precocious sexual development in immature males.

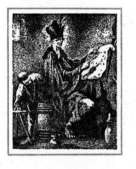

EUNUCH
(after GOYA)

Eunuchs (G., *eunouchos*, guarding the couch) are produced by removal of the testicles or castration. Before puberty, this results in complete deficiency of male sex hormone before normal mature development has taken place. Hence, prepuberal eunuchism is characterized by any combination of the following: immature, unaggressive demeanor; puerile facial development; underdeveloped larynx with high-pitched voice; scanty or absent hair on the face, pubic and arm-pit regions, and on the body in general; narrow flat chest; undeveloped muscles; excess fat on the hips, abdomen and breasts; disproportionately long arms and legs; undeveloped reproductive organs with infantile penis, scrotum, etc.; loss of sexual desire or libido; and impotence.

Actual removal of the testicles is not necessary in order for such changes to take place. Occasionally, during childhood, testicular infections (e.g., mumps), injuries or congenital deficiency of unknown origin, result in varying degrees of androgenic deficiency, known as hypogonadism, sexual juvenilism or eunuchoidism (eunuch + G., *eidos*, resemblance).

If the testicles are removed surgically or destroyed by disease after puberty, the resulting body changes are not as pronounced as are those in prepuberal eunuchism, because normal male development has already taken place. There are, however, marked nervous and emotional instability, diminished sense of energy, tendency to mental depression, hot flushes, diminished libido, and impotence.

The eunuch and the eunuchoid states have varying degrees of androgenic deficiency occurring at different periods of life. Both are amenable to therapy with male sex hormone.

The male sex hormone is formed in the testicles. Other substances with androgenic activity of lesser degree have been obtained from the urine of men, bulls and steers, as well as from the urine of women and pregnant cows.

Not only have androgens been obtained from female sources, but estrogens have also been extracted from male sources, such as the urine of men, steers and stallions. Stallion urine, in particular, is an extremely rich source, containing twice as much estrogen as the urine of pregnant mares. It seems probable that there is a balance between androgen and estrogen in the male, similar to that existing between estrogen, progesterone and androgen in the female.

PHYSIOLOGY

The main action of male sex hormone is exerted on the male accessory sex organs (penis, scrotum, seminal vesicles and prostate) and secondary sex characteristics (depth of voice, distribution of hair, muscular and skeletal development, mental attitudes and interest in the opposite sex).

In immature male animals, injections of androgen cause precocious development of the sexual organs and instincts; and reverse the regression and atrophy of the sexual organs in castrated animals. These effects are duplicated in the human male. In normal adult animals, the male hormone causes considerable enlargement of the sexual organs.

The developmental effect of androgens on the atrophied organs of castrated animals is used as a method of bio-assay. For instance, the growth of the seminal vesicles and prostate in castrated rats, and the restoration of ejaculatory function in castrated mice have been utilized as tests. A more reliable method

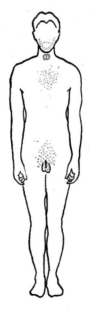

MALE SECONDARY SEX
CHARACTERISTICS

61

is the capon comb test. Androgen is administered to capons (castrated roosters) conforming to certain specifications. Originally, the capon unit was described as the amount which, injected per day for five days, yielded an average of 5 mm. increase in length of the combs of brown leghorn capons. At present, the increase in size of the capon's comb is compared with that obtained with a known standard and the result is expressed in terms of the standard in International Units.

In addition to its effects on the growth and development of the sexual organs, male sex hormone stimulates the functions of erection and ejaculation and increases sexual desire. This has been observed not only in immature and castrated animals, but also in hypogonadal adults.

Besides primordial action on the male reproductive system, the male sex hormone has other biologic effects:

1. It influences the blood supply and pigmentation of the entire human skin, and has a beneficial effect on certain skin diseases occurring in late middle life (and possibly related to androgenic deficiency), characterized by dryness, fissuring, itching and eczema.

2. It affects muscular and skeletal development, muscle tone, endurance and recovery after exertion.

3. It increases the resistance of the nervous system to fatigue, it relieves such symptoms of testicular failure as nervous irritability, insomnia, apprehension, and restores effective mental ability not only in concentration but also in the fulfilling of social and economic responsibilities.

4. It may influence peptic ulcer, which is thought by some to be due to a disturbed pituitary-gonad relationship.

5. It causes an increase in the size and weight of the kidneys, and has been employed experimentally to protect the kidneys from toxic substances, such as mercuric chloride.

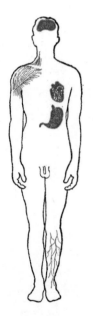

EXTRA-GENITAL
TISSUES INFLUENCED
BY TESTOSTERONE

6. It relieves pain in certain forms of heart disease such as angina pectoris.

7. It improves the peripheral circulation in certain arterial diseases (e.g., arteriosclerosis; Buerger's disease).

8. It has an effect on the blood similar to that of the adrenal cortical hormone, desoxycorticosterone, favoring the retention of sodium, chlorides and water, and the excretion of potassium.

9. It inhibits breast function, and has been found to suppress lactation and to reduce the masses in chronic cystic mastitis (lumpy breasts).

10. It inhibits the growth of fibroids in the human uterus, suppresses uterine bleeding, and, in adequate dosage, may temporarily suppress all cyclic activity in women.

11. It inhibits the pituitary production of gonadotropic hormone (which is probably the mode of action when male hormone is employed in gynecology).

12. It is associated synergistically with estrogen to maintain normal hormonal balance in males; it also neutralizes the effects of estrogens in females.

POTENCY AND UNITS

The dosage of testosterone, the pure, crystalline male sex hormone, is expressed in milligrams. Since the relatively inactive hormones have been virtually discarded by clinicians, cross-reference to unit equivalents is not necessary as it still is with estrogens. For determinations of extracts and body fluids, such as the urinary androgen excretion, the capon comb method of assay may be used. For purposes of comparison, it may be noted that 1 mg. testosterone ⇌ 70 to 100 I.U.

MALE SEX HORMONE PREPARATIONS

Testosterone, the primary androgenic hormone is available in the free form, esterified as the propionate, and as the methyl derivative.

Pure crystalline testosterone in the form of a compressed tablet for subcutaneous implantation is ORETON-F.

The propionate, in ampules for intramuscular injection, is ORETON.

The methyl derivative, in tablets for oral use and in ointment for local application, is available as ORETON-M. Approximately three to five milligrams of the latter, when given orally, have the clinical effect of one milligram of ORETON by injection. All the clinical effects of male sex hormone therapy may be achieved with ORETON-M by mouth.

All ORETON preparations permit effective male sex hormone therapy by different routes. ORETON by injection represents the dosage form of greatest effectiveness for prolonged high activity as may be required for intensive initial treatment. ORETON-F is suitable for prolonged substitution therapy as required in the treatment of hypogonadism and the male climacteric. ORETON-F Pellets may be implanted by means of the Kearns Pellet Injector or by making a simple surgical incision and placing the hormone in subcutaneous pockets. The use of pellets should be preceded in all cases by ORETON injections intramuscularly to determine the necessary maintenance dose. ORETON-M, containing the only orally effective androgen, may be used to supplement injection therapy, and is especially valuable when injections are not feasible. The use of ORETON-M in ointment form serves to supplement injection or oral therapy during the intensive course.

CHAPTER ELEVEN

MALE SEX HORMONE THERAPY

Of the various physiological effects of the male hormone, some are utilized in clinical medicine and others are still in the experimental stage. Androgen therapy depends, in general, on the following effects of the hormone:

1. *Developmental action on the reproductive organs.* In this connection, male hormone is administered not only to castrates, but also in hypogonadism of all types, including eunuchoidism, the male climacteric and impotence. In castrates, therapy which is substitutive, is necessarily lifelong. In other cases, initially high dosage is gradually reduced, and, depending on the effects obtained, eventually may be discontinued.

2. *Correction of estrogen-androgen imbalance.* This action, or possibly that on the pituitary, is utilized in the treatment of benign prostatic hypertrophy. The neutralizing effect of androgen upon estrogen is also employed in gynecologic disorders.

3. *Inhibition of pituitary hormones.* The use of the male sex hormone in gynecology, e.g., suppression of lactation, and certain patients with the menopausal syndrome, depends not only on the direct negating action of androgen on estrogen, but primarily on the suppression of pituitary hormones, such as prolactin and the gonadotropins.

PRINCIPAL INDICATIONS IN THE MALE

Hypogonadism

SYMPTOMS

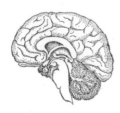

The symptoms of eunuchoidism or hypogonadism resemble closely those seen in complete castration or true eunuchism and may be grouped as follows:

1. Vasomotor: flushes, headaches.
2. Nervous: fatigability, emotional instability.
3. Secondary sex characteristics: effeminate appearance, immature and retiring behavior, high-pitched voice, sparse or absent hair on face, pubic region and chest.
4. Skeletal development: usually long arms and legs, broad hips.
5. Genital apparatus: genital organs of infantile proportions, absent libido, impotence.

When functional deficiency develops during adult life, the anatomical characteristics may regress only slightly, but the nervous and vasomotor symptoms are more prominent. They include depression, fatigability, impaired mental powers, lack of ambition, flushes, sweats, sexual indifference and impotence.

EFFECTS OF TREATMENT*

Male sex hormone therapy with ORETON has resulted in improvement even in long-standing cases. Among the effects are:

1. Increase in size of the sexual organs: penis, scrotum, seminal vesicles and prostate.

---

*See Plate VIII.

2. Development of the secondary sex characteristics: increase of hair on the pubis, body, arms, legs and face; deepening of the voice.

3. Increased libido and potency, and, in some cases, the performance of the sex act for the first time.

4. Development of masculine psychological outlook with increased aggressiveness, maturity and self-confidence.

5. Increase in muscular development and gain in weight.

6. Increase in strength, vitality and energy, and decrease in fatigability.

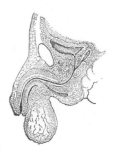

DOSAGE

Advanced dosage is necessary for rapid anatomic and functional effects. Treatment may be instituted with 25 mg. ORETON three or more times a week. When clinical improvement is manifest, the dosage may be gradually diminished, first by reducing the number of injections, and then by employing 10 mg. ORETON injections two or more times weekly, supplemented by one or two 10 mg. tablets of ORETON-M daily. Maintenance dosage depends upon the requirements of the individual patient, and may be furnished as two 10 mg. ORETON-M Tablets daily, or as ORETON-M Ointment applied nightly to non-hairy portions of the skin. After maintenance dosage has been established by any of the above forms of hormone, ORETON-F Pellets implanted subcutaneously will be found most convenient for continuous treatment.

The Male Climacteric

With declining testicular function in middle age, there develops a syndrome termed the "male climacteric" generally resembling the menopausal syndrome of women. Because of the underlying hormonal insufficiency, the male climacteric is amenable to treatment with male hormone, which serves to restore the hormone deficiency and to abolish the troublesome symptoms.

SYMPTOMS

Symptoms are mainly nervous and sexual, and resemble those seen in the female climacteric. They include emotional instability, irritability, fatigability, despondency, diminished mental powers, general lassitude, and even flushes and sweats in severe cases. There may be a vague sense of slackening of physical and mental force, diminution of interest and loss of concentration for normal social and economic activities. In some cases, there may be a weakening or loss of sexual potency, or a lack of normal interest in sex life.

TREATMENT

Treatment restores physical and mental powers as well as emotional equilibrium. Mental quiet replaces the previous irritability and instability, and, as energy increases, there is increased interest in business and social life. In those cases where there has been diminished libido and potency, there is a return of normal sexual satisfaction.

DOSAGE

Initial treatment may consist of three injections weekly of ORETON, 25 mg. for several weeks, after which 10 mg. ORETON may be injected two or three times weekly. Oral therapy may then be substituted, using ORETON-M Tablets of 10 mg. three to five times daily in the most pronounced cases; or in the average patient, two to three times daily. Maintenance therapy varies from one patient to another; it usually may be furnished as one or two ORETON-M Tablets of 10 mg. daily, or as 2 to 4 mg. ORETON-M Ointment daily, or by implantation of ORETON-F Pellets.

Impotence

The problem of impotence and its treatment is exceedingly complicated and difficult. In frank hypogonadism, as in castrates, impotence is usually associated with diminished libido. However, in the type of impotence most frequently encountered, sexual desire is present, but the proper accomplishment of the sexual act is difficult or impossible, usually because of inadequate penile erection, as regards either rigidity of the organ or duration of the process, or both.

The mechanism of penile erection depends upon several elements, much as links in a chain; one such link is evidently the presence of an adequate amount of male sex hormone. Other links are psychic factors, general state of health and energy, and local factors such as infections. These are of the greatest importance, and weakness of any one link may result in relative or complete sexual impotence. Weakness of the endocrine link is amenable to therapy with the male sex hormone.

If the patient has an obviously underdeveloped genital apparatus (hypogonadism), then it is clear that his impotence is merely part of the picture and will respond to endocrine therapy. Impotence as a manifestation of the male climacteric, due to functional male hormone deficiency, likewise will respond. In the case of the young or middle-aged adult male, where there is no objective sign of testicular deficiency and no indication of any other organic cause that might be responsible for the impotence, a therapeutic test with male sex hormone may be of value.

DOSAGE

Treatment consists of 25 mg. ORETON by injection three times weekly for two or three weeks. If the patient responds satisfactorily, dosage may be adjusted to a lower level, employing injection, oral or inunction therapy as desired. In some cases, a higher level of therapy may be necessary.

Benign Prostatic Hypertrophy

The direct effect of enlargement of the prostate is urinary obstruction of a variable degree, giving rise to a number of symptoms, frequently referred to as prostatism. Prostatism includes urination during the night or nocturia (L., *nox*, night + *urina*, urine), increased frequency of urination during the day, difficulty in starting the urinary stream and dribbling of urine. As the prostatic hypertrophy progresses, the bladder empties less and less completely, the urine may become infected, and ascending urinary infection may result. Complete urinary retention occurs in advanced cases.

NORMAL SIZE OF PROSTATE (*white*). ENLARGED PROSTATE (*red*) TO SHOW PRESSURE ON NEIGHBORING STRUCTURES.

EFFECTS OF TREATMENT

Since prostatic hypertrophy occurs during late middle age or old age when testicular function is declining, male hormone deficiency has been suggested as a causative factor, possibly by disturbing estrogen-androgen balance.

Administration of ORETON preparations results in marked improvement of the urinary symptoms, with diminution in frequency of urination, particularly during the night, increase in force of the urinary stream, and decrease in dribbling. There is greater ease in starting the stream, and the bladder empties more completely. These effects are probably due to improved bladder muscle tone.

In addition, male sex hormone considerably improves the patient's general state of health, probably by its constitutional tonic effects. If surgery should prove necessary for prostatism, pre-operative endocrine treatment improves the patient's health and resistance, making him a better operative risk. Post-operative male sex hormone treatment also helps speed recovery. Reports indicate that the hormone markedly reduces the complications and the duration of convalescence.

DOSAGE

The general dosage range is 25 mg. ORETON by injection three times weekly, supplemented on the alternate days by two to three 10 mg. tablets of ORETON-M. After four to six weeks, dosage may be gradually reduced, depending on the response obtained. Maintenance therapy may be conveniently given as two 10 mg. ORETON-M Tablets daily. If prostatectomy is indicated, ORETON may be given in the initial full dosage for two weeks before and after operation.

Dwarfism

Recently, clinical investigators have shown that dwarfism and retarded growth when associated with hypogonadism in boys may be influenced favorably by male sex hormone provided it is given before the epiphyses of the long bones have united. Dosage for accelerating growth is 10 mg. to 25 mg. ORETON two times weekly for 3 to 6 months. A rest period for a month or two between courses is indicated to prevent excessive genital development.

Precautions

Since the male sex hormone is a physiological substance normally present in the body, it does not produce any undesirable side effects in adult males, other than priapism. It should be administered with discretion to elderly patients in whom undue activity, sexual or otherwise, is undesirable.

PRINCIPAL INDICATIONS IN WOMEN

Androgens normally occur in women and may be utilized in the treatment of certain gynecological disorders. The mode of action appears to depend mainly on an inhibitory effect on the pituitary gland and on a neutralizing effect on excessive estrogen.

Functional Uterine Bleeding

When meno-metrorrhagia is excessive and resistant to usual methods of therapy, it may be rapidly arrested by treatment with the male sex hormone, thus relieving the worry and anxiety of the patient, preparatory to substitution and stimulative hormone therapy. Appropriate dosage is 25 mg. ORETON by injection every second day for three doses or more as required. The mode of action is probably that of neutralization of excessive estrogen.

About one week after control of the uterine hemorrhage, therapy with corpus luteum hormone (PROLUTON) may be begun as outlined on page 58, to be followed, if desired, with pregnant mare serum (ANTERON), see page 81.

Dysmenorrhea

Intractable dysmenorrhea not responding to either follicular hormone or corpus luteum hormone therapy may be relieved by intermittent use of male sex hormone. Suitable dosage is 25 mg. ORETON by injection once weekly, or three ORETON-M Tablets of 10 mg. daily during the latter half of the cycle. To avoid abolition of menstruation the dosage of ORETON should not exceed 300 mg. per month.

After-pains

It has been observed that patients given male sex hormone shortly after delivery do not experience after-pains. Suitable dosage is 10 mg. ORETON injected at the end of labor and repeated, if desired, in eight hours. Lactation is not affected by male hormone given at this time and in this dosage.

Control of Lactation

The action of the male sex hormone in suppressing lactation is based on the inhibition of the pituitary lactogenic hormone. Limitation of fluids, breast-binders, ice packs, and purgatives are unnecessary. Treatment, which is best begun on the third day after delivery, consists of 25 mg. ORETON by injection twice daily for two days.

Breast Engorgement

Small doses of ORETON, such as 10 mg. daily for two or three days, may be given to relieve painful engorgement of the breasts after delivery *without impairing* milk production. It is important that nursing of the child be continued regularly when only relief is desired without suppression of milk.

Chronic Cystic Mastitis

An indication which is still in the experimental stage is chronic cystic mastitis characterized by breast pain, heaviness and lumps. For relief, injections of 25 mg. ORETON twice weekly have been advocated. Here, too, the mechanism is probably by neutralization of estrogenic hormone effects. Dosage should not exceed 300 mg. ORETON per month.

Menopausal Syndrome

While the menopausal syndrome usually responds very satisfactorily to estrogenic hormone therapy, there are certain cases, especially when associated with excessive uterine bleeding, which are best treated with male sex hormone. Dosage is 10 mg. ORETON by injection twice weekly.

Precautions

Male sex hormone therapy in women has no untoward effects except when dosage exceeds approximately 300 mg. per month; with excessive dosage, undesirable effects may be noted, as growth of facial hair, enlargement of the clitoris, and deepening of the voice. These are transitory, and disappear after treatment is discontinued or dosage reduced.

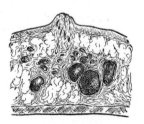

CHRONIC CYSTIC MASTITIS, (AFTER HOMANS, *Textbook of Surgery*)

CHAPTER TWELVE

THE GONADOTROPINS

As members of the hormonal symphony, the sex glands are subject to control by the conductor, the pituitary gland. Among the several hormones secreted by the anterior pituitary are the gonadotropic hormones, or gonadotropins which stimulate the development of the ovaries and testes. These, in turn, secrete the sex hormones that stimulate the growth of the sexual organs and determine the secondary sex characteristics of the individual. Moreover, as shown in previous chapters, the sex hormones themselves, have an inhibitory effect on the pituitary gland, suppressing or reducing the production of gonadotropins. It is thus apparent that sexual development and function depend on a delicate balance between the gonadotropic hormones and the various sex hormones. The stimulating effect of the gonadotropins on the gonads is utilized in medicine, either alone, or in combination with sex hormone therapy.

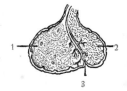

1. *pars anterior*
2. *pars posterior*
3. *pars intermedia*

CROSS-SECTION OF
PITUITARY GLAND

The direct relationship between the anterior pituitary and the gonads has been experimentally demonstrated in an interesting and striking manner. For instance, it was shown that removal of the pituitary gland before sexual maturity caused the sexual organs to remain permanently in an infantile state. When pituitary extract was subsequently administered, this was prevented. Likewise, when pituitary tissue was transplanted into an immature animal, precocious sexual development resulted.

THE GONADOTROPIC FACTORS*

Subsequent investigation showed that there are two distinct gonadotropic hormones.

1. The follicle-stimulating hormone, which causes growth of the ovarian follicle (producing follicular hormone) in woman; and development of the tubules of the testis and production of spermatozoa in man.

2. The luteinizing hormone, which causes growth of the corpus luteum (producing corpus luteum hormone) in woman; and development of the interstitial tissue of the testis (producing male sex hormone) in man.

These experiments were carried on with extracts of pituitary glands from various animals, particularly the horse, the sheep and the pig. Because of the technical difficulties encountered in preparing the extracts, which frequently contained other substances with undesirable side effects, different sources of gonadotropic hormones were sought.

Human Pregnancy Urine

In 1928, Aschheim and Zondek discovered in the urine of pregnant women, gonadotropic substances which were termed prolans. Animal experimentation showed that these could be divided into two fractions: (1) Prolan A, which has an action similar to the follicle-stimulating hormone (abbreviated FSH); and (2) Prolan B, which has an action similar to the luteinizing hormone (abbreviated LH). At first, the prolans were thought to be identical with the gonadotropins obtained from the anterior pituitary itself. Later, it was decided that they were produced in the chorionic portion of the placenta, and were therefore called chorionic gonadotropins.

*See Plates III and VII.

76

Gonadotropic hormone is present in the urine of normal non-pregnant women in very small amounts, and in larger amounts in menopausal urine. During pregnancy, there is a marked increase in the production of the hormone, which is excreted mainly in the urine. The presence of detectable amounts of gonadotropic hormone in the urine is therefore characteristic of pregnancy. (Large amounts of gonadotropic hormone are also produced in patients with certain rare tumors.)

If human pregnancy urine is injected into animals, and gonadotropins are present, corpora lutea and "blood spots" are produced in the ovaries.

The Aschheim-Zondek test for pregnancy in the human female (commonly abbreviated as AZ test) is performed on female mice, takes 4 days for its completion, and is accurate in about 98% of cases. More rapid results may be obtained by using rabbits (Friedman test) or the South African toad, *Xenopus laevis* (Xenopus test).

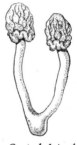

Control Animal

Pregnant Mare Serum

A new source of gonadotropic hormone was discovered in 1930 by Cole and Hart in the blood serum of pregnant mares. This gonadotropin is found in the mare's urine in very small amounts, and appears to have a different action from the gonadotropin obtained from human pregnancy urine.

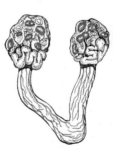

Positive Test
(pregnancy)

ASCHHEIM-ZONDEK TEST

CHEMISTRY

The chemical structure of the gonadotropic hormones, which have been prepared in very pure form, has not yet been exactly determined. They appear to be proteins with molecular weights between 60,000 and 80,000 and to belong to the group of glycoproteins (combinations of protein with carbohydrate).

Gonadotropic hormones may be extracted from various

sources. Those obtained from the anterior pituitary itself are called pituitary gonadotropins; those obtained from other sources, such as urine or blood serum are termed "anterior-pituitary-like" hormones because their action is similar to but not exactly identical with that of the pituitary gonadotropins.

The chief sources of gonadotropic hormone are human pregnancy urine (abbreviated PU) and pregnant mare serum (abbreviated PMS) also called equine gonadotropin. Other sources are urine from menopausal women (MU), urine from castrate women (CU) and urine from patients with certain types of rare uterine or testicular tumors. Gonadotropic activity is also exhibited by extracts from such non-animal sources as brewer's yeast and green leaves.

PHYSIOLOGY

The physiological effects of the gonadotropins vary with the source, probably because these preparations contain different amounts of the follicle-stimulating factor and the luteinizing factor. Pregnancy urine gonadotropin, for instance, consists essentially of the luteinizing factor, while menopausal urine and castrate urine consist mainly of the follicle-stimulating factor. Pregnant mare serum contains both factors, with a preponderance, however, of the follicle-stimulating factor.

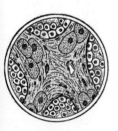

INTERSTITIAL TISSUE
OF TESTIS

It has been found that pregnancy urine gonadotropin produces descent of the testes in patients in whom descent has failed to take place normally. The exact mechanism, though obscure, is probably by stimulation of the interstitial tissue of the testis with production of male hormone which acts on the various anatomical structures involved to effect the descent.

Pregnant mare serum gonadotropin which, of all the pituitary-like preparations most closely resembles the pituitary gonadotropins, produces gonadal stimulation not only in animals, but also in the human. The artificial production of ovulation in women, followed by normal corpus luteum development, has been achieved with pregnant mare serum hormone, and some investigators have reported a high percentage of pregnancies following its use in long-standing sterility attributed to ovarian failure.

POTENCY AND UNITS

Since the gonadotropic hormones are not crystalline compounds but natural extractives of great chemical complexity, their potency must be determined by bio-assay and expressed in units rather than in milligrams.

The assay is usually done on immature rats, and is based on the production of a direct gonadotropic effect, e.g., increase in ovarian weight or presence of luteinization, or an indirect effect on the accessory organs, e.g., increase in uterine weight or production of an estrous vaginal smear. The results are compared with the International standards prepared from the urine of pregnant women and from the serum of pregnant mares, and are expressed in International Units.

PREPARATIONS

The gonadotropic hormone from pregnant mare serum (PMS) is available as ANTERON. The ampule of ANTERON contains the dry stable substance in tablet form, and each tablet-ampule is provided with a solution-ampule containing distilled water for preparing the solution at the time of administration. The freshly prepared ANTERON solution is usually administered intramuscularly.

CHAPTER THIRTEEN

GONADOTROPIC HORMONE THERAPY

The aim of therapy in the female with pregnant mare serum hormone (ANTERON) is the stimulation of the ovary, and ripening of the graafian follicles with resulting ovulation followed by corpus luteum formation. In the male, ANTERON also has been shown to exert a stimulating action on the testicular tubules with production of spermatozoa.

The chief therapeutic indication for pregnancy urine hormone (PRANTURON) is in the treatment of undescended testes. It has also proved effective in functional uterine bleeding, which, however, is better treated with pregnant mare serum. Recently, PRANTURON, administered to dwarfed hypogonad boys resulted in unusually rapid increase in height.

PRINCIPAL CLINICAL INDICATIONS

Female Sterility

Sterility, due to either partner, is present in at least twelve per cent of marriages. Two-thirds of all causes of sterility are found in the female.

Most sterile women have no obvious organic defects and no impairment of normal sexual development. These cases may require ovarian stimulation with gonadotropic hormone from pregnant mare serum (ANTERON). Ovulation is not the only possible result of such treatment. There is also stimulation of the endocrine (both estrogenic and luteal) functions of the ovary with improvement in the reproductive organs in general, particularly in rendering the endometrium more receptive to the implantation of a fertilized ovum.

However, organic causes, such as uterine fibroids or inflammation of the neck of the uterus or of the fallopian tubes, are not amenable to endocrine therapy and require other measures. Infertile women with symptoms of hypogonadism are best treated first with estrogenic hormone. The administration of PROGYNON results in the development of the sexual organs including the uterus, and renders them more receptive to the stimulating effect of gonadotropin therapy.

Amenorrhea

In amenorrhea due to anterior pituitary hypofunction, ANTERON may be administered in five daily injections of 400 International Units beginning about four days after the arbitrarily calculated menstrual date. For some patients 800 units daily are required and a sixth dose of 2000 International Units may be given for even greater stimulation.

Functional Uterine Bleeding

After uterine bleeding has been controlled with ORETON or with PROLUTON (either alone or combined in full cyclic therapy with PROGYNON), gonad-stimulating therapy with ANTERON may be instituted in an attempt to restore normal cyclic activity.

ANTERON is often of value in meno-metrorrhagia, a condition seemingly contrasting completely with amenorrhea. Here, too, there is diminished ovarian follicular activity with lack of ovulation and of luteinization and persistence of a proliferative type of endometrium.

Daily injections of 400 or 2000 I.U. for five days beginning on the eighth day of the cycle.

Male Sterility

Since one-third of all causes of sterility are present in the male, examination of the husband is important in the treatment of infertility. If there is no organic disease, resulting, for instance, from previous infection of the testicles or of the vasa deferentia, examination of the sperm may reveal such abnormalities as oligospermia, azoospermia and necrospermia.

Male Hypogonadism

Cases of hypogenitalism and delayed puberty due to pituitary hypofunction have been successfully treated with administration of pregnant mare serum, particularly when preliminary treatment with male hormone has been given. In men ANTERON is administered three times weekly in injections of 400 I.U. for a period of 2 to 3 months. It is then discontinued for 2 months and a new course inaugurated.

In cases of sterility associated with hypogonadism, it is possible to produce a normal adult level of sexual development, libido and potency with ORETON. Spermatogenesis is not affected by the male sex hormone.

Undescended Testicles

Correction of cryptorchidism is important not only because undescended testicles are usually sterile, but also because of the tendency to atrophy and tumor-formation, the propensity to hernia, and the unhappy psychologic effect on the young boy's outlook. It also appears from experimental

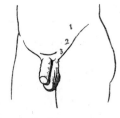

1. abdominal
2. high inguinal
3. low inguinal

SITES OF
UNDESCENDED TESTES

work that endocrine function of the testes may suffer.

Therapy with gonadotropic hormone from human pregnancy urine (PRANTURON) produces descent of cryptorchid testes in a large percentage of cases. Moreover, the use of this hormone, by distinguishing between those patients in which descent is prevented by anatomical factors and those in which it is not, makes it possible to determine which patient will require surgical operation. When surgery does become necessary, preliminary gonadotropic therapy is of help by partially enlarging the parts involved.

PRANTURON should be employed after the age of seven years and before puberty. It is given in doses of 150 to 750 I.U., three times a week. While the response is frequently very prompt, a course of treatment of six to twelve weeks may be necessary.

In a certain proportion of cases, possibly half, cryptorchidism is merely a part of the general picture of hypogonadism. In cases of this type, the preliminary administration of ORETON 25 mg. by injection two times weekly is usually desirable as an adjunct to PRANTURON therapy.

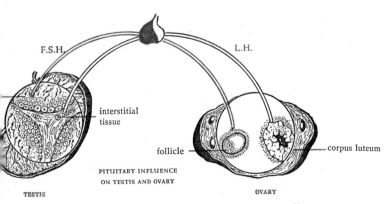

F.S.H.

L.H.

interstitial tissue

follicle

corpus luteum

PITUITARY INFLUENCE
ON TESTIS AND OVARY

TESTIS

OVARY

PACKAGE INFORMATION

PROGYNON-B, α-estradiol benzoate, *ampules* of 1 cc. containing 500, 1000, 2000, 6000 and 10,000 R.U. (0.083, 0.166, 0.333, 1.0 and 1.666 mg.) ; boxes of 3, 5, 6, 50 and 100 ampules.

PROGYNON-DP, α-estradiol dipropionate, *ampules* of 1 cc. containing 0.2, 0.5, 1.0, 2.5 and 5.0 mg.; boxes of 6 and 50 ampules.

PROGYNON-DH TABLETS, α-estradiol in tablet form, containing 0.1, 0.2 and 0.5 mg. per *tablet;* boxes of 30, 60 and 250 tablets.

PROGYNON-DH SOLUTION, α-estradiol in solution for oral administration by drop dosage, containing 3600 R.U. per cc. or 60 R.U. per drop as delivered by dropper (furnished) ; *bottles* of 10 cc.

PROGYNON-DH OINTMENT, α-estradiol for inunction, containing 360 R.U. per gram in *tubes* of 50 grams, and 1800 R.U. per gram in *tubes* of 25 and 50 grams, for local application. (One inch of ointment as squeezed from tube represents approximately one gram.)

PROGYNON-DH SUPPOSITORY, α-estradiol in glycerinated gelatin vaginal *suppositories,* in juvenile, 480 R.U. (0.04 mg.) ; and adult, 480 R.U. (0.04 mg.) and 4800 R.U. (0.4 mg.) sizes; boxes of 10 and 30.

ORETON, testosterone propionate, *ampules* of 1 cc. containing 5, 10 and 25 mg.; boxes of 3, 6 and 50 ampules.

ORETON-M TABLETS, methyl testosterone, in *tablet* form, containing 10 mg.; boxes of 15, 30 and 100 tablets.

ORETON-M OINTMENT, methyl testosterone for inunction, containing 2 mg. of hormone per gram, ($2\frac{1}{2}$ inches of ointment as squeezed from tube represents approximately 4 mg.) ; *tubes* of 50 grams.

ORETON-F PELLETS, pure compressed testosterone pellets, for subcutaneous implantation containing 75 mg. of hormone; boxes containing 1 and 3 vials; one sterile pellet per vial.

PROLUTON, corpus luteum hormone, (progesterone) in oil for injection; *ampules* of 1 cc. containing 1, 2, 5 and 10 mg.; boxes of 3, 6 and 50 ampules.

PRANONE, orally effective progestin (anhydrohydroxy-progesterone) *tablets* for oral administration containing 5 and 10 mg.; boxes of 20, 40, 100 and 250 tablets.

ANTERON, gonadotropic hormone from pregnant mare serum (PMS), *ampules* of dry hormone containing 400 I.U. in boxes of 6 and 50 ampules with diluent; and 2000 I.U. in boxes of 3 ampules with diluent.

PRANTURON, chorionic gonadotropic hormone from pregnancy urine (PU), *ampules* of dry hormone containing 150 I.U., in boxes of 3 and 10 ampules with diluent; and 750 I.U., in boxes of 6 and 50 ampules with diluent.

INDEX

Abortion; definition of, 53; due to corpus luteum deficiency, 53; habitual, 53, 56; prevention of, 53, 54, 56; therapy of, 56; threatened, 53, 56

After-pains; treatment with male sex hormone, 73

Alpha-estradiol; benzoate, advantages of, 39; chemistry of, 13; comparative potency of, 37; constitutional effects of, 34, 40; dipropionate, advantages of, 39; esters of, 14, 38; history of, 17; nasal spray, 38, 50; ointment, 14, 39; physiology of, 33; potency of, 13, 37; preparations of, 14, 38; structural formulae of, 13; suppositories, 38, 48; tablets, 14, 38; therapy, 40; see estrogens

Amenorrhea; definition of, 45; etiology of, 45; in hypo-ovarianism, 44; primary, 45; secondary, 45; therapy of, with estrogens, 45, with pregnant mare serum, 45

Androgens, 60; biologic effects of, 62; chemistry of, 15; comparative potency of, 63; deficiency of, 60; definition of, 15; history of, 20; physiology of, 61; potency and units of, 63; preparations of, 64; structural formulae of, 15; therapy, see male sex hormone; types of, 16

Androsterone; in urine, 15

Angina pectoris; effect of male sex hormone in, 63

Anhydrohydroxy-progesterone; see corpus luteum hormone, progestins

Anterior pituitary; hormones of, 32; interrelationship of gonads and, 31, Plates III, VII; inhibitory effect of sex hormones and, 31; secondary sex characters and, 32

ANTERON; see gonadotropins

Arthritis; endocrine factor in, 43; menopausal, 43

Aschheim-Zondek test, 77

Aspermia; definition of, 30

Atrophic rhinitis; estrogens and, 50

Azoospermia; definition of, 30

Breast; anatomy of, 27; cystic mastitis, 73; development of, with estrogens, 48; hypoplasia, 44, 48

Capon test, 62

Corner-Allen Rabbit Unit; definition of, 51

Corpus luteum hormone, 51; chemistry of, 14; comparative potency of, 15; history of, 19; physiology of 51; potency of, 15, 54; preparations of, 54; structural formulae of, 14; therapy, 55

Cryptorchidism; definition of, 28; therapy of, with luteinizing hormone, 82, 83

Cystic mastitis; therapy of, with male sex hormone, 63; see breast

Dehydro*iso*androsterone; in urine, 15

Dysmenorrhea; definition of, 36; etiology of, 57; functional, 46, 57; in hypo-ovarianism, 44; organic, 46; therapy of, with corpus luteum hormone, 55, 57, with estrogens, 44, 46, with male sex hormone, 57, 72; types of, 46

Endocrine glands; function of, 8; interrelationship of, 9, Plates III, VII; types of, 8

Endocrinology; history of, 9, 17

Endometrium; definition of, 26; gravid phase, 51; influence of hormones on, 35, Plate III; proliferative, 35; secretory, 35, 51

Epididymis; anatomy of, 28, Plates V, VI; function of, 28

Esters; of alpha-estradiol, 14, 38; of testosterone, 15, 64

Estriol; comparative potency of, 37, 38; in urine, 13

Estrogens; actions of, 40; chemistry of, 13; comparative potency of, 37; deficiency of, 40; definition of, 13; esters of, 14, 38; estrogen therapy of amenorrhea, 45, arthritis, 43, breast development, 48, dysmenorrhea, 46, frigidity, 47, functional uterine bleeding, 58, 59, gonorrheal vaginitis, 27, 48, hypertension, 43, lactation, 40, 49, menopause, 41, 42, menstrual cycle, 35; general function of, 34; history of, 17; physiology of, 33; potency and units of, 37; preparations, 14, 38; structural formulae of, 13; therapy, 41; types of, 16

Estrone; comparative potency of, 37; in urine, 13

Eunuchism, adult; androgenic deficiency in, 60; characteristics of, 60, 66; etiology of, 60; prepuberal, 60; therapy of, 65

Necrospermia; definition of, 30
Nervousness; male sex hormone and, 62; see male climacteric
Neuroses; menopausal, 50

Oligomenorrhea; definition of, 36
Oligospermia; definition of, 30
Ovaries; anatomy of, 25, 26, Plates I, II
Ozena; estrogens and, 50
ORETON; see androgens, testosterone, and male sex hormone
ORETON-F; ORETON-M; see androgens, testosterone, and male sex hormone

Penis; anatomy and function of, 29, Plates V, VI; see impotence
Peptic ulcer; effect of male sex hormone on, 62
Pituitary, 9; see anterior pituitary
Placenta; anatomy and function of, 52
PRANONE; see corpus luteum hormone, progestins
PRANTURON; see gonadotropins and luteinizing hormone
Pregnancy; physiology of, 51; tests for, 77; therapy during, with corpus luteum hormone, 53; therapy of, disturbances, 49; uterine motility in, 53; nausea and vomiting, 49; see abortion
Pregnancy toxemia; high blood pressure and, 59; therapy of, with corpus luteum hormone, 59
Pregnant mare serum hormone (PMS); see follicle-stimulating hormone
Premenstrual tension, 58
Progestins; definition of, 14; chemistry of, 14; history of, 19; structural formulae of, 14; potency of, 15; types of, 16
PROGYNON-B; see alpha-estradiol, estrogens
PROGYNON-DH Tablets, Solution, Ointment, Suppositories; see alpha-estradiol, estrogens
PROGYNON-DP; see alpha-estradiol, estrogens
Prolactin, 40; see lactation
Prolan A; chorionic gonadotropin, 76
Prolan B; chorionic gonadotropin, 76
PROLUTON; see corpus luteum hormone, progestins
Prostate; anatomy and function of, 29, 70, Plate V

Prostatic hypertrophy; male sex hormone deficiency in, 70; therapy of, with male sex hormone, 71
Psychoneuroses; in menopause, 50
Psychoses; in menopause, 41
Rat Unit (R.U.); definition of, 34, 37
Reproductive system, 24, 25; anatomy of female, 25, 26, Plates I, II; anatomy of male, 28, Plates, V, VI

Seminal vesicles; anatomy and function of, 29, Plates V, VI
Sex characters; at puberty, male and female, 23; hypogonadism, male and female, 25; secondary, 25, 31, 34, 45; sex glands and, 23
Sex hormones; chemistry, 11
Sexual infantilism, 44; see hypogonadism
Skin; male sex hormone and, 62
Spermatozoa, 29, 30, 82
Sterility; and relation to follicle-stimulating hormone, 80; etiology of, 46; female, 80; in hypo-ovarianism, 44; male, 82
Steroids; chemistry of, 12; definition of, 11
Stilbestrol, 22
Testes; anatomy of, 28, Plates V, VI; function of, 28
Testosterone; chemistry of, 15; comparative potency of, 16; definition of, 15; esters of, 15, 64; history of, 20; ointment, 16, 64; physiology of, 61; potency of, 63; preparations of, 64; propionate, advantages of, 15; structural formulae of, 15; tablets, 16, 64; therapy, 65; see androgens and male sex hormone
Testosterone propionate; see testosterone
Uterine motility; inhibition of, 55; in pregnancy, 53
Uterus; anatomy of, 26, Plates I, II; bleeding from, 55; effect of hormones on, 51
Vagina; anatomy of, 27, Plate II
Vaginal smear; for bio-assay, 34; for diagnoses in menopause, 42, 43
Vas deferens; anatomy of, 28, Plates V, VI; function of, 28
Vulvovaginitis; juvenile, 48; treatment of, 48

This book was designed by L. W. FROHLICH AND COMPANY, INC.
and printed by THE GEORGIAN PRESS, INC.

HO-20